keto Baking Made Easy

An ABC guide for beginners about the ketogenic lifestyle. Try this fantastic recipe book, your weighing machine will be grateful!

Author: **Carolyn Taylor**

Table Of Contents

INTRODUCTION

The ketogenic diet, colloquially called the keto diet, is a popular diet containing high amounts of fats, adequate protein and low carbohydrate. It is also referred to as a Low Carb-High Fat (LCHF) diet and a low carbohydrate diet.

It was primarily formulated for the treatment of epilepsy that did not respond to medications for the disease.

The diet was originally published in 1921 by Dr. Russell Wilder at the Mayo Clinic. Dr. Wilder discovered that putting epileptic patients on a fast helped to reduce the frequency of the symptoms. At the time of its publication, there were few other options available for the treatment of epilepsy.

The ketogenic diet was widely used for the next several decades in treating epilepsy both in children and adults. In several epilepsy studies, about 50% of patients reported having at least 50% reduction in seizures.

However, the arrival of anticonvulsant drugs in the 1940s and afterward relegated the ketogenic diet to an "alternative" medicine. Most health, as well as patients, found it a lot easier to use the pills compared to adhering to the strict ketogenic diet. It was subsequently ignored in the treatment of epilepsy by most specialists.

In 1993, a renewed interest in the ketogenic diet was sparked by Hollywood producer Jim Abrahams. Abraham had his 2 years old

1

son, Charlie, brought to the Johns Hopkins Hospital for epilepsy treatment. Charlie experienced rapid seizure control within days of using the ketogenic diet.

Jim Abrahams created the Charlie Foundation in 1994 which helped to revive research efforts. His production of the TV movie called "First Do No Harm" starring Meryl Streep also helped to greatly promote the ketogenic diet.

To understand why this Ketogenic Diet can be so effective at burning fat you have to look at how your body normally operates. The body's preferred source of fuel is carbohydrates and is very effective at metabolizing carbohydrates to use for fuel. Because of this fact, your body actually craves carbohydrates on a regular basis which usually leads to us overeating them. When the body eats too many carbohydrates than it can process and use, it breaks them down, converts them and stores some of them as fat for later use. If your body does not have a source of carbohydrates to use for energy, it will utilize the next available source. If you severely limit the number of carbohydrates that you eat and instead replace them with fat, your body will go through a process and adjustment that will allow it to metabolize the fat for energy as well. In addition, once the body begins to use fat as fuel it will be much easier for it to metabolize stored fat as fuel thereby helping to speed up existing fat loss.

The meals were designed to provide the body with the right amount of protein it needs for growth and repair. The calculation of the amount of consumed calories was done to provide adequate amounts that will be able to support and maintain the proper weight necessary for the child's height and weight.

CHAPTER ONE

INTRODUCTION TO KETOGENIC DIET

For the best diet to rapidly burn fat using the body's natural metabolism, consider a ketogenic diet plan. Nutrition has the strongest effect on the body's production of important hormones, which regulate metabolism and allow the body to burn fat for energy and retain muscle mass, with little need for excessive exercise.

WHAT IS A KETOGENIC DIET PLAN?

It is a diet that causes the body to enter a state of ketosis. Ketosis is a natural and healthy metabolic state in which the body burns its stored fat (producing ketones), instead of using glucose (the sugars from carbohydrates found in the Standard American Diet - SAD).

Metabolically speaking, ketogenic foods are very powerful. The amazing benefit is that these foods are also delicious, natural whole foods that are extremely healthy for you.

When you eat a very low amount of carbs your body gets put into a state of ketosis. What this means is your body burns fat for energy? How low of an amount of carbs do you need to eat in order to get into ketosis? Well, it varies from person to person, but it is a safe bet to stay under 25 net carbs. Many would suggest that when you are in the "induction phase" which is when you are actually putting your body into ketosis, you should stay under 10 net carbs.

If you aren't sure what net carbs are, let me help you. Net carbs are the amount of carbs you eat minus the amount of dietary fiber. So if on the day you eat a total of 35 grams of net carbs and 13 grams of dietary fiber, your net carbs for the day would be 22. Simple enough, right?

UNDERLYING CONCEPTS OF THE KETOGENIC DIET

The classic ketogenic diet has a "fat" to a "combination of protein and carbohydrates" ratio of 4:1.

The general daily calorie breakdown of the ketogenic diet is as follows:

60-80% of calories from fat

20-25% from proteins

5-10% from carbohydrates

The ratio of the foods in a ketogenic diet is formulated to help the body induce and maintain a state of ketosis.

However, the ketogenic landscape has expanded considerably both in its application and implementation. While the classical ketogenic diet is still extensively used today, it has now formed the basis for the development of several alternative ketogenic protocols.

Ketogenic diets encourage the intake of about 20 to 50 grams of carbohydrates per day. Protein consumption is moderate and mostly depends on factors such as the gender, height and activity levels of the individual. Essentially, the overall calorie of the diet is balanced primarily based on the amount of consumed fat.

Many diets promoted are calorie restriction diets. They help you lose weight, but, most of the weight is in the form of water and muscle. Little fat stores are broken down. Here is the problem with a calorie restrictive eating program. Your metabolism gets slower because your body begins to think it is starving and must slow down the process of losing calories. A slow metabolism equals slower weight loss and faster weight gain!

The cyclical ketogenic diet restricts carbohydrates. By restricting carbohydrates, but, maintaining caloric consumption, your body will have only one option of fuel consumption. That is fat; which is what ketosis is. You are essentially turning on your fat burning machine. Ketones are sent out of your body and fat loss becomes profound. How does this happen? The largest internal organ in your body is the key player. Your liver. The liver has the job of converting fat into ketones. These ketones are then excreted out of the body, weight/fat loss. This is a natural process.

Ketones are created in the liver and are an efficient source of energy for the body. Fatty acids that are broken down from body fat are created in the liver as these ketones. Ketones can only be made present when there is a lack of of sugar and glucose in the body. Carbohydrates contain both of these substances. It will always be difficult to lose weight on a high carbohydrate based diet. On the ketogenic diet, the amount of sugar and glucose is reduced to the point where they are no longer the primary source of fuel to be burned in the bloodstream.

We should take a moment and talk about a couple of myths surrounding the ketogenic diet and whether it is healthy long term. Our bodies can perform in the state of ketosis and be healthy. This state of ketosis is a natural occurrence when the body is not using sugar and glucose. The human body has no problem operating in this state naturally. In other words, it is safe to burn fat!!

How do you know if you are in a fat-burning state? A simple walk to the drug store can answer that quickly. You can use ketone testing strips to check your level of ketosis. Simply capture a urine sample on the strips and check for a color change. The magic color to look for is a pink to purple result. Check the color scale to see your ketone level and where you are in the fat burning zone.

The use of these strips will be your source of the level of ketones being released. This is the gauge by which you will know if you are properly keeping your carbohydrate intake to the necessary level to facilitate ketosis. Don't worry if you are not at the dark purple level. Different people have different levels. Just watch the scale and if you are losing weight, you are pretty much ok!

HISTORY OF KETOGENIC DIET

In 1921, the Mayo Clinic was on the verge of a massive breakthrough. For centuries, physicians attempted to treat epilepsy through different means of dietary remedies with fasting being one of the most successful treatments. But one doctor suggested that the effects of fasting could be captured in a diet. More specifically, the Ketogenic Diet.

The first modern use of starvation as a treatment for epilepsy was recorded by a pair of Parisian physicians, Gulep and Marie, in 1911 (Guelpa & Marie, 1911). They treated 20 children and adults with epilepsy and reported that seizures were less severe during treatment, but no specific details were given. The United States contemporary accounts of fasting were also recorded early in the 20th century: the first was a report on a patient of an osteopathic physician, Dr. Hugh W. Conklin, of Battle Creek, Michigan; and the second concerned Bernarr Macfadden (Freeman et al., 1994). Macfadden was a physical fitness guru/cultist and publishing genius of the early part of the 20th century.

He advised readers how to develop themselves physically, how to maintain their health, and how to cope with illness. Each issue of his magazine, Physical Culture, carried articles about sickly men and women who became healthy, strong, and beautiful through proper diet and exercise. By the end of World War I, the magazine's circulation had reached 500,000. Macfadden claimed that fasting for 3 days to 3 weeks could alleviate and cure just about any disease, including epilepsy. He had become nationally recognized, and in 1931 tried to ingratiate himself with a presidential candidate,

Franklin D. Roosevelt, as part of a strategy to be appointed as the first Secretary of Health (Wilkinson, 1997).

Dr. Conklin began as an assistant to Macfadden and adopted his method of fasting to treat various ailments. It was Dr. Conklin's practice of fasting to treat epilepsy and the results, which drew the attention of another pioneer in epilepsy study, H. Rawle Geyelin, an endocrinologist at New York Presbyterian Hospital. Dr. Geyelin first reported at the American Medical Association Convention in 1921 his experience with fasting as a treatment of epilepsy (Geyelin, 1921). Dr. Geyelin was the first to document the cognitive improvement that could occur with fasting. Attending Dr. Geyelin's presentation were Drs. Stanley Cobb and W.G. Lennox of Harvard.

The success of Dr. Conklin's results with fasting quickly spread and by 1941 it had achieved prominence in the textbook of Penfield and Erickson on epilepsy from the Montreal Neurologic Institute (Penfield & Erickson, 1941). In the early 1920s, Drs. Cobb and Lennox at Harvard Medical School began studying the effects of starvation at a treatment for epilepsy. They were the first to note that seizure improvement typically occurred after 2–3 days. Lennox documented that the control of seizures occurred through a change of body metabolism and that simple absence of food or dearth of carbohydrate in the body forced the body to burn acid-forming fat.

In 1921, two pivotal observations were made. Woodyatt noted that acetone and beta-hydroxybutyric acid appear in a normal subject by starvation or a diet containing too low a proportion of carbohydrate and too high a proportion of fat (Woodyatt, 1921). Concurrently, Dr. Wilder at the Mayo Clinic proposed that the benefits of fasting could be obtained if ketonemia was produced by other means (Wilder, 1921). Wilder proposed that a ketogenic diet (KD) be tried in a series of patients with epilepsy. He suggested that the diet should be as effective as fasting and could be maintained for a much longer period of time.

Wilder subsequently reported on patients treated with the ketone-producing diet at the Mayo Clinic and coined the term "ketogenic diet." Subsequently, Peterman at the Mayo Clinic reported the calculation of KD similar to that used today: 1 g of protein per kilogram of body weight in children, 10–15 g of carbohydrates per day, and the remainder of the calories in fat (Peterman, 1925). Peterman documented the importance of teaching caregivers management of the diet before discharge, individualization of the diet, and close follow-up. Peterman also noted improvements in behaviour and cognitive effects that accompanied the KD.

These initial reports were rapidly followed by reports from Talbot et al. from Harvard and McQuarrie and Keith at the Mayo Clinic. The use of the KD was recorded in almost every comprehensive textbook on epilepsy in children that appeared between 1941 and 1980. Most of these texts had full chapters describing the diet, telling how to initiate it, and how to calculate meal plans (Wheless, 2004). Throughout the 1920s and 1930s, the KD was widely used.

In his 1972 textbook, Livingston, at Johns Hopkins Hospital, reported on the results of the diet in over 1,000 children with epilepsy that he had followed over the prior decades (Livingston, 1972). He suggested that 52% had complete control of the seizures and an additional 27% had improved control.

When Merritt and Putnam discovered diphenylhydantoin in 1938, the attention of physician and researcher shifted focus from the mechanism of action and efficacy of the KD to new antiepileptic drugs. A new era of medical therapy for epilepsy had begun and the KD fell by the wayside. In an effort to make the classic KD more palatable, Dr. Peter Huttenlocher, at the University of Chicago, in 1971 introduced a medium-chain triglyceride oil diet, allowing less restriction of other foods.

As new antiepileptic drugs became available, the KD was used less and less. After the introduction of sodium valproate, it was believed that this branched-chain fatty acid would treat children previously placed on the diet to treat the seizures of Lennox–Gastaut syndrome and the diet could no longer be justified. Pediatric neurologists were led to believe that rationally designed antiepileptic drugs were the hope for the future. Fewer children were placed on the KD, resulting in fewer dietitians trained in the use of the diet. A shortage of properly trained dietitians meant that the KD was often implemented without correct calculation, leading to the perception that the diet was ineffective. The use of the KD has always been dependent on

11

public perception.

MODERN ERA OF THE KETOGENIC DIET

Use of the KD decreased greatly and PubMed listed only two to eight publications per year from 1970 to 2000. However, this changed dramatically when the KD received national media attention when NBC-TV's Dateline aired a program on the treatment. Corresponding with this was a dramatic spike in PubMed publications averaging over 40 a year since then. This television program was based on the true story of Charlie, a 2-year-old boy with intractable generalized seizures, who presented out of desperation to Johns Hopkins Hospital for treatment. He was seen by Dr. Freeman and Ms. Millicent Kelly (the same dietitian who had worked with Dr. Livingston) and initiated on the KD.

He quickly became seizure-free and The Charlie Foundation was formed by his father. This foundation disseminated informational videos for parents and instructional videos for physician's and dietitians about the KD. It also helped fund the initial publication of The Epilepsy Diet Treatment: The Introduction to the Ketogenic Diet (Freeman et al., 1994).

The Foundation supported the first multicenter prospective study of the efficacy of the KD (Vining et al., 1998), and in 1997, Charlie's father directed the film "First Do No Harm" starring Merryl Streep, which aired on national TV.

The KD has experienced a reemergence in recent years and modern clinical studies have established the treatment as significantly effective (Freeman et al., 1998). The KD is now is available in over 45 countries (Kossoff & McGrogan, 2005). However, physician perception still greatly affects when this therapy is utilized by pediatric neurologists.

Two recent expert opinion surveys, one conducted in the United States and one conducted in Europe, revealed that the KD was the next-to-the-last or last choice for treatment of almost all childhood epilepsies. In addition, a recent survey of practising child neurologists also ranked the KD as a therapy they typically used last, with many not using it at all (Mastriani et al. 2008). Much work still needs to be done to improve the perception of the utility of the KD, a treatment that compares favourably with other new treatments that have been introduced to treat childhood epilepsy.

THE DANGER OF HIGH-FAT DIETS

After smoking, a high-fat diet is the second most lethal habit. According to a report published in the Journal of the American Medical Association, smoking causes 400,000 deaths a year. High-fat diets cause 300,000. Several more highly publicized social evils are comparatively small problems: alcohol (100,000 deaths), guns (35,000), auto accidents (25,000) and drug abuse (20,000). These statistics in no way minimize the tragedies of alcoholism, murder or drug addiction. But they provide a perspective on what is really like killing us. If this sounds a bit extreme, consider the dangers of dietary fat and judge for yourself.

1.   High Blood Pressure.

High blood pressure is a major risk factor for heart disease and stroke. A high-fat diet contributes to this condition because it adds extra pounds. As weight increases, the heart must work harder to pump blood through all the extra tissue. As the heart's effort increases, so does blood pressure.

2.   Diabetes.

Diabetes contributes to an estimated 250,000 deaths a year. It involves an inability to metabolize blood sugar because of problems with the pancreatic hormone, insulin. In Type I (insulin-dependent) diabetes, the pancreas stops producing insulin. In more common Type II (non-insulin-dependent) diabetes, typically associated with obesity, insulin production may be normal, but food intake overwhelms the body's ability to process it.

3.   Arthritis.

Dietary fat contributes to the most common form of arthritis, osteoarthritis because excess weight subjects the major joints to extra weight and tear. A high-fat diet also appears to increase the risk of rheumatoid arthritis (RA), the most serious and potentially

14

crippling form of joint disease. Several studies suggest that a low-fat diet relieves RA symptoms.

4.   Stroke.

Stroke is the nation's third leading cause of death, claiming 144,000 lives a year. There are two major types of stroke, one caused by bleeding in the brain (hemorrhagic), the other by blockage of an artery there (ischemic). About 75 percent of strokes are ischemic, and the vast majority of ischemic strokes are caused by cerebral thrombosis - blockage of a brain artery by a process similar to heart attack, involving atherosclerosis and plaque rupture.

5.   Obesity.

Many people use obese as a synonym for fat, but it has a more precise medical definition - a weight 20 percent heavier than what is recommended for one's height and build. Anyone who is 35 percent overweight faces a risk of premature death 50 percent greater than average. Obesity is a risk factor for heart disease, several cancers, high blood pressure, diabetes, and arthritis. It is a problem only in countries with a high-fat diet. In addition to being hazardous to health, obesity is also an economic handicap, since obese people earn less money than those who are slimmer.

6.   Heart Disease.

The nation's leading cause of death, heart disease kills 720,000 Americans a year, most as a result of heart attacks. About one American in four has some form of heart disease. Heart disease results from a process called atherosclerosis, which is directly linked to dietary fat. Fatty foods are high in cholesterol and free radicals, which are oxygen molecules that have lost an electron and become highly reactive. As they circulate in the blood, they snatch electrons away from other molecules, sometimes grabbing them from the cells that line artery walls. The microscopic injuries that free radicals inflict begin a decades-long process that eventually narrows the arteries with cholesterol-rich deposits called plaques. Sometimes plaque rupture, spilling their contents into the blood. If a plaque ruptures in one of the coronary arteries that nourish the heart, its debris can cause complete blockage. Without food and oxygen to nourish its hard-working cells, part of the heart dies. That's a heart attack.

USES AND BENEFITS OF THE KETOGENIC DIET

When using a ketogenic diet, your body becomes more of a fat-burner than a carbohydrate-dependent machine. Several researches have linked the consumption of increased amounts of carbohydrates to development of several disorders such as diabetes and insulin resistance.

By nature, carbohydrates are easily absorbable and therefore can be also be easily stored by the body. Digestion of carbohydrates starts right from the moment you put them into your mouth.

As soon as you begin chewing them, amylase (the enzymes that digest carbohydrate) in your saliva is already at work acting on the carbohydrate-containing food.

In the stomach, carbohydrates are further broken down. When they get into the small intestines, they are then absorbed into the bloodstream. On getting to the bloodstream, carbohydrates generally increase the blood sugar level.

This increase in blood sugar level stimulates the immediate release of insulin into the bloodstream. The higher the increase in blood sugar levels, the more the amount of insulin that is release.

Insulin is a hormone that causes excess sugar in the bloodstream to be removed in order to lower the blood sugar level. Insulin takes the sugar and carbohydrate that you eat and stores them either as glycogen in muscle tissues or as fat in adipose tissue for future use as energy.

However, the body can develop what is known as insulin resistance when it is continuously exposed to such high amounts of glucose in the bloodstream. This scenario can easily cause obesity as the body tends to quickly store any excess amount of glucose. Health conditions such as diabetes and cardiovascular disease can also result from this condition.

Keto diets are low in carbohydrate and high in fat and has been associated with reducing and improving several health conditions.

One of the foremost things a ketogenic diet does is to stabilize your insulin levels and also restore leptin signalling. Reduced amounts of insulin in the bloodstream allow you to feel fuller for a longer period of time and also to have fewer cravings.

Medical Benefits Of Ketogenic Diets

The application and implementation of the ketogenic diet has expanded considerably. Keto diets are often indicated as part of the treatment plan in several medical conditions.

1.   Epilepsy

This is basically the main reason for the development of the ketogenic diet. For some reason, the rate of epileptic seizures reduces when patients are placed on a keto diet.

Pediatric epileptic cases are the most responsive to the keto diet. There are children who have experience seizure elimination after a few years of using a keto diet.

Children with epilepsy are generally expected to fast for a few days before starting the ketogenic diet as part of their treatment.

2. Cancer

Research suggests that the therapeutic efficacy of the ketogenic diets against tumor growth can be enhanced when combined with certain drugs and procedures under a "press-pulse" paradigm.

It is also promising to note that ketogenic diets drive the cancer cell into remission. This means that keto diets "starves cancer" to reduce the symptoms.

3. Alzheimer Disease

There are several indications that the memory functions of patients with Alzheimer's disease improve after making use of a ketogenic diet.

Ketones are a great source of alternative energy for the brain especially when it has become resistant to insulin. Ketones also provide substrates (cholesterol) that help to repair damaged neurons and membranes. These all help to improve memory and cognition in Alzheimer patients.

4. Diabetes

It is generally agreed that carbohydrates are the main culprit in diabetes. Therefore, by reducing the amount of ingested carbohydrate by using a ketogenic diet, there are increased chances for improved blood sugar control.

Also, combining a keto diet with other diabetes treatment plans can significantly improve their overall effectiveness

5. Gluten Allergy

Many individuals with gluten allergy are undiagnosed with this condition. However, following a ketogenic diet showed improvement in related symptoms like digestive discomforts and bloating.

Most carbohydrate-rich foods are high in gluten. Thus, by using a keto diet, a lot of the gluten consumption is reduced to a minimum due to the elimination of a large variety of carbohydrates.

6. Weight Loss

This is arguably the most common "intentional" use of the ketogenic diet today. It has found a niche for itself in the mainstream dieting trend. Keto diets have become part of many dieting regimen due to its well acknowledged side effect of aiding weight loss.

Though initially maligned by many, the growing number of favorable weight loss results has helped the ketogenic to better embraced as a major weight loss program.

Besides the above medical benefits, ketogenic diets also provide some general health benefits which include the following.

7. Improved Insulin Sensitivity

This is obviously the first aim of a ketogenic diet. It helps to stabilize your insulin levels thereby improving fat burning.

8. Muscle Preservation

Since protein is oxidized, it helps to preserve lean muscle. Losing lean muscle mass causes an individual's metabolism to slow down as muscles are generally very metabolic. Using a keto diet actually helps to preserve your muscles while your body burns fat.

9. Controlled Ph And Respiratory Function

A ketoc diet helps to decrease lactate thereby improving both pH and respiratory function. A state of ketosis therefore helps to keep your blood pH at a healthy level.

10. Improved Immune System

Using a ketogenic diet helps to fight off aging antioxidants while also reducing inflammation of the gut thereby making your immune system stronger.

11. Reduced Cholesterol Levels

Consuming fewer carbohydrates while you are on the keto diet will help to reduce blood cholesterol levels. This is due to the increased state of lipolysis. This leads to a reduction in LDL cholesterol levels and an increase in HDL cholesterol levels.

12. Reduced Appetite and Cravings

Adopting a ketogenic diet helps you to reduce both your appetite and cravings for calorie rich foods. As you begin eating healthy, satisfying, and beneficial high-fat foods, your hunger feelings will naturally start decreasing.

13. Helps Squash Migraines

• **Decreased Migraine Frequency**

In recent studies, scientists have found that the ketogenic diet significantly reduced the frequency of migraines in 90% of patients. This completely dwarfs the effects of migraine drugs.

• **Glutamate Inhibition**

Glutamate is found in both epilepsy and migraine patients. Medications that work in epilepsy (anti-seizure drugs) also block glutamate production. These drugs have been used to treat migraines as well. Since about 500 BC, ketones have worked to help prevent seizures, but the ketogenic diet has only been popular for the last century.

• **Processed Food**

Processed foods are bad for you, especially if you suffer with migraine. "Food-like products" are filled with preservatives, chemicals, and other triggers that could be affecting your migraine symptoms. Any diet that removes those processed foods, including the ketogenic diet, would be a good step to controlling migraine symptoms.

- **Saturated Fats**

Several studies have debunked the great saturated fat myth. There are plenty of saturated fats (and other healthy fats) in a ketogenic diet, which has been found to reduce bad cholesterol and help the body produce serotonin and vitamin D, both of which help prevent migraines.

- **Hunger vs. Weight Management**

Hunger is a major migraine trigger, so is weight gain/obesity. Some studies have found that weight gain and/or obesity increases the risk of migraines by 81%. Ketones help reduce hunger, while controlling insulin problems, promoting weight loss, and regulating glucose levels in the blood.

Weight loss and sugar control are well-known benefits to adding MCT or coconut oil to your diet. Now, as you can see, they will help control migraines by helping you feel nutritionally satisfied, more energetic, improve cognitive functioning, and lose fat.

- **Oxidative Stress**

A recent study found that oxidative stress is tied to migraine triggers. In response to these findings, a new migraine medication has come out which blocks the peptide released during oxidative stress. This drug also prevents glutamate release, another migraine trigger. You don't need to depend on medication, however. A ketogenic diet will do both for you, which indicates that ketones can not only treat migraine symptoms, but also determine the root cause.

- **MCT Oil**

Research has found that Alzheimer's patients respond favorably to MCT (medium-chain triglyceride) oil, especially concerning memory recall. Like Alzheimer's, migraine patients have white-matter brain lesions on their scans. Research in both diseases has found that ketones may help increase metabolism in the brain, even when oxidative stress and glucose intolerance is present.

Our minds and bodies need glucose and/or ketones to function and survive. We store about 24 hours' worth of sugar in our bodies, but we'd all die of hypoglycemia if not for the ketones. Metabolizing ketones from fat leaves our body in a healthy state of ketosis.

Migraines indicate that the brain is not metabolizing glucose into energy properly, so the logical response would be to add ketones. In addition to migraine pain symptoms, the ketogenic diet can help reduce:

• Brain fog

• Oxidative stress

• Brain Lesions

CHAPTER TWO

TYPES OF KETOGENIC DIETS

Ketogenic Diet is divided into three types and depending on one's daily calorie needs, the percentage differs. Diets are often prepared on a ratio level such as 4:1 or 2:1 with the first number indicating the total fat amount in the diet compared to the protein and carbohydrate combined in each meal.

1.   Standard - SKD

The first diet is the Standard or the SKD and is designed for individuals who are not active or lead a sedentary lifestyle. The meal plan limits the dieter to eat a net of 20-50 grams of carbohydrates. Fruits or vegetables that are starchy are restricted from the diet. In order for the diet to be effective, one must strictly follow the meal plan. Butter, vegetable oil and heavy creams are used heavily to replace carbohydrates in the diet.

2.   Targeted - TKD

The TKD is less strict than the SKD and allows one to consume carbohydrates though only in a certain portion or amount which will not impact the ketosis that one is currently in. The TKD diet helps dieters that perform some level of exercise or workout.

3. Cyclical - CKD

The CKD is preferable for those who are into weight training or do intensive exercises and not for beginners as it requires the person undergoing the diet to stick to an SKD meal plan for the five days in a week's time and eating/loading up on carbohydrates on the next two days. It is important that dieters follow the strict regimen to ensure that their diet is successful.

KETOGENIC AND FOOD TO AVOID

The three main macronutrients that are relatable to a keto diet are fats, proteins, and carbohydrates. All three of these nutrients have different effects on ketosis from their digestion and have consequent effects on blood glucose and hormones.

1. Fats are 90% ketogenic and 10% anti-ketogenic, due to the small amount of glucose that is released in the conversion of triglycerides.

2. Proteins are typically ranked at 45% ketogenic and 58% anti-ketogenic since insulin levels rise from over half of the ingested protein being converted to glucose.

3. Carbohydrates are of course 100% anti-ketogenic, as they raise both blood glucose and insulin.

PROTEIN

Protein is vitally important in a ketogenic diet, but it's also a tricky nutrient. If we don't eat enough protein, we lose muscle mass. You might be thinking "well I can just eat all the meat I can to overdose on the stuff." Well, that would be pretty delightful, but the massive amounts of proteins would raise the glucose levels in our bloodstream.

As you saw, protein is 46% ketogenic and 54% anti-ketogenic, meaning that too much of the stuff will knock us out of ketosis. We have to fall between narrow ranges in our protein intake: enough to not lose muscle mass, but not too much to knock us out of ketosis.

This narrow range is quite hard to determine, as it differs from person to person. Some have reported trouble maintaining keto if they eat excessive protein in a single day, or if they eat too much protein in 1 sitting. Others have 1.2g of protein per pound of body weight and have no problems transitioning and staying in ketosis.

This may also be in relation to the amount of exercise you do, as glycogen depletion, will allow carbohydrates to be used up quicker. That being the case, the suggested protein intake depends on your lean body mass and what your activity levels are like.

• Sedentary: 0.8g of protein per pound of lean body mass.
• Lightly Active: 0.8 – 1.0g of protein per pound of lean body mass.
• Highly Active: 1.0 – 1.2g of protein per pound of lean body mass.

Healthy Ketogenic Proteins

Animal proteins (meat, fish, etc.) have very little, if any, carbs. You can consume them in moderate amounts as needed to control hunger. Overall, choose fattier cuts of meat rather than leaner ones. For example, chicken thighs and legs are preferable to chicken breasts because they contain much more fat.

• Grass-fed beef and other types of fatty cuts of meat, including lamb, goat, veal, venison and other game. Grass-fed, fatty meat is preferable because it's higher in quality omega-3 fats — 0 grams net carbs per 5 ounces

• Organ meats including liver — around 3 grams net carbs per 5 ounces

• Poultry, including turkey, chicken, quail, pheasant, hen, goose, duck — 0 grams net carbs per 5 ounces

• Cage-free eggs and egg yolks — 1 gram net carb each

• Fish, including tuna, trout, anchovies, bass, flounder, mackerel, salmon, sardines, etc. — 0 grams net carbs per 5 ounces

Foods to Avoid:

It is always best to purchase grass-fed, organic and free-range humanely raised animals. Avoid the hormone-fed animals, especially with rBST.

Also, when buying processed meat products, you should check the carbohydrate content as they might have been added through the extenders and fillers used. You need to also avoid meats that have been cured with sugar or honey.

FATS

Even though the ketogenic diet is known for the high amounts of fat eaten, dietary fats have a pretty minimal effect on ketosis. In the end, fat intake will determine how much body fat is being used for fuel.

Since fats are 90% ketogenic and only 10% anti-ketogenic, we can get away with significant amounts of fat intake. Yes, the glycerol from triglycerides produce glucose but think of it regarding the number of grams you eat. If you eat, say, 160g of fats in 1 day – that is only 16g of glucose.

Since fats are mostly consumed over the entire day and not just in 1 sitting, your body will be using that glucose without you even noticing it's there. The only time in the day we deviate from a consistent fat intake is after a workout. Fats slow down the digestion process and will slow the absorption of the protein you intake after your workout, so they're not recommended.

Healthy Ketogenic Fat

Healthy fats include saturated fats, monounsaturated fats and certain types of polyunsaturated fats (PUFAs), especially omega-3 fatty acids. It's best to include all types in your diet, with an emphasis on saturated fats, especially compared to PUFAs.

•   MCT oil, cold-pressed coconut, palm fruit, olive oil, flaxseed, macadamia and avocado oil — 0 net carbs per tablespoon

•   Butter and ghee — 0 net carbs per tablespoon

•   Lard, chicken fat or duck fat — 0 net carbs per tablespoon

Foods to Avoid:

When consumed in large amounts, omega-6 fatty acids can cause inflammation in the body. This can just be as damaging as the increase in sugar consumption.

Also, seed or nut-based oil should be avoided as they are also high in omega-6 that can have inflammatory effect.

Some of the polyunsaturated fatty acids and nut-based oil to avoid include:

Canola oil, Corn oil, Cottonseed oil, Flax oil, Grapeseed oil, Peanut oil, Safflower oil, Sesame oil, Soybean oil, Sunflower oil, Vegetable oil, Walnut oil

Hydrogenated and Trans Fats

Trans fat are the most inflammatory of all fats. Several studies have noted that foods containing trans fats increase the risk of developing heart disease and cancer.

Also, avoid mayonnaise and commercial salad dressing and if unavoidable, check their carbohydrate content and include in it your carbohydrate counts.

CARBOHYDRATES

As one of the most restricted nutrients on a ketogenic diet, the carbohydrate has the biggest effect on ketosis. The general rule is to consume no more than 30g of carbs a day if on an SKD.

As carbohydrates are processed, they are converted almost gram to gram into glucose when entering the bloodstream. Here, the glucose has a number of different things that it can do. It will either be burned up immediately for fuel, stored as glycogen in the muscles or liver or if excess carbohydrates are consumed, it will be stored in fat cells.

Healthy Ketogenic Carb

Carbohydrates are divided into two categories: simple and complex. Sugar is a simple carb and starch and fiber are complex carbs. Whether a food is classified as a simple or complex carbohydrate depends on how many sugar molecules it contains.

There are three nutrients (sugar, starch and fiber) that make up carbohydrates. These three nutrients can be found in combination with a single food. It is rare to find a food in nature that contains just one of the three. For example, sweet potatoes are a complex carbohydrate commonly referred to as a starchy vegetable, but they also contain fiber and sugar. Likewise, berries are a simple carbohydrate and contain sugar, but they're also a great source of fiber.

Whether a carbohydrate is classified as simple or complex should not determine whether that carb is good or bad. Instead, you should look at how much sugar, fiber and starch are in that particular food, and what kind of effect it will have on your blood sugar levels.

Foods to Avoid:

Some of the common carbohydrates to avoid include the following grains and grain products:

Amaranth, Barley, Bread crumbs, Bread, Buckwheat, Bulgur, Cakes, Cookies, Corn chips, Cornbread, Cornmeal, Crackers, Grits, Kashi, Muffins, Oatmeal, Oats, Pancakes, Pasta, Pies, Polenta, Popcorn, Pretzels, Quinoa, Rice, Rolls, Rye, Sorghum, Spelt, Tarts, Tortillas, Tricale, Waffles, Wheat.

VEGETABLES

Vegetables are the main carbohydrate sources in a ketogenic diet. Also, a lot of vegetables that grow underground are starchy and contain a lot of carbohydrates.

You should limit your consumption of Brussels sprout, green beans and pumpkin as the carbs can add up quickly.

However, you should avoid the following vegetables:

Carrots, Corn, Green peas, Leeks, Parsnips, Potatoes, Squash, Sweet potatoes, Yams, Yuca

TROPICAL FRUITS

Avoid most tropical fruits including mango, papaya, and pineapple as they are usually high carbohydrates. Also avoid 100 percent fresh juice since most of them are often high in sugars.

SUGARS AND SWEETENERS

Sugar is a very rich source of glucose and must therefore be avoided. Also, sugar is known in forms like brown sugar, white, castor and icing sugar. Sugar can also be an ingredient in processed foods.

Barley malt, Beet sugar, Brown sugar, Cane juice, Cane syrup, Caramel, Carob syrup, Coconut sugar, Corn syrup, Date sugar, Fruit juice concentrate, Fruit syrups, Malt syrup, Maltose, Maple syrup,

Molasses, Panela, Panocha, Rice syrup, Sorghum, Tapioca syrup, Treacle, Turbinado sugar, White sugar.

NUTS

Moderate amounts of nuts and seed are allowed on the ketogenic diet. Nuts and seed are rich in protein, fats, and carbohydrates. The total fat, protein and carbohydrate content of the nut varieties should be checked and added to the total daily calorie calculation.

Roasted nuts and seeds are the best. Anything that may cause harm or interfere with ketosis in the body has been removed from them through the roasting process.

Nuts should be used mostly as a snack

Almonds, Macadamia, and Walnuts are some of the best

Some nuts have high content of omega-6 fatty acid which can cause inflammation in the body

However, they can hold some people back from their goals. If your weight loss is purely your purpose of using the ketogenic diet, then it would be advisable to remove nuts and seeds to improve your results.

Almonds, Brazil nuts, Hazelnuts, Pine nuts, Macadamia nuts, Pecans, Pili nuts, Pumpkin seeds, Sesame seeds, Sunflower seeds, Walnuts

HERBS AND SPICES

After some time on the ketogenic diet, the foods may start to become boring. Adding spices to your meals can however help to spice things up. You can add fresh and dry spices to your meals and even beverages so that they become more enticing and exciting to the palate.

Spices and fresh herbs are some of the most nutrient-dense foods on the planet you can eat. Adding spices to your meal doesn't only add more flavors to the meals but also offer a lot of various health benefits to your body.

Spices contain carbohydrates thus you should ensure to add them to your daily carbohydrate count. Also, endeavor to check the labels of pre-made spice mixes for their accurate carbohydrate content as they usually contain added sugars.

Salt also enhances flavors. It is best you chose high quality sea salt instead of traditional table salt. Unprocessed salts such as Celtic or Himalayan sea salt provide you with more than eight trace minerals that your body need to perform optimally.

Anise, Annatto, Basil, Bay leaf, Black pepper, Caraway Cardamom, Cayenne pepper, Celery seed, Chervil, Chili pepper, Chives, Cilantro, Cinnamon, Cloves, Coriander, Cumin, Curry, Dill, Fenugreek, Galangal, Garlic, Ginger, Lemongrass, Licorice, Mace, Marjoram, Mint, Mustard seeds, Oregano, Paprika, Parsley,

Peppermint, Rosemary, Saffron, Sage, Spearmint, Star anise, Tarragon, Thyme, Turmeric, Vanilla beans

BEVERAGES

Using a low carbohydrate diet like the ketogenic diet has a diuretic effect on the body. Carbohydrates draw water to them which cause water retention in the body. However, the reduced carbohydrate intake in a ketogenic diet leads to a lot water loss as less water is retained in the body and more is excreted.

This diuretic effect can easily lead to dehydration. Therefore you need to drink a lot of water - well above the recommended intake of 8 glasses - when you are on a ketogenic diet. This will help you to reduce the risk of bladder pain and urinary tract infections.

Besides water, you can add other types of beverages like coffee and teas to help keep your hydrated throughout the day. Both of these do not significantly affect the ketosis state.

However, the added substances like sugar and milk might affect the ketosis state. As a result, it would be best to avoid the sugar completely and use either full cream or artificial sweeteners together with your coffee or tea.

Another way to increase your beverage intake is to make vegetable juice by combining varieties of the approved vegetable types. You can also use a power smoothies or protein shakes instead of a fruit smoothies as the fruits contain sugars (fructose) that can kick you out of ketosis.

Below are some additional beverages you can be consuming to help keep you hydrated:

Unsweetened almond milk, Unsweetened cashew milk, Unsweetened coconut milk, unsweetened hemp milk, Green tea, Herbal tea, Organic caffè Americano (espresso with water), Mineral water.

IMPORTANT KETOGENICS MISTAKE TO AVOID

Almost everyone makes mistakes! While mistakes usually aren't a big deal, in the keto world they can be a very bad thing mentally for you. When you get started on keto you expect to see results because you see all of the amazing results that others are achieving and you want the same thing.

When those things don't happen because of mistakes it can be very frustrating and lead you to believe that keto just isn't for you.

Here are 5 common Keto mistakes to avoid

1.   Not Enough Fats

One of the hardest adjustments for people to make when starting keto is making sure they consume enough fats.

You probably not used to consuming the amount of fat daily and it can be a struggle to find foods that have the fats you need.

However, on keto, if you want to lose fat, you need to consume fat so that means hitting your daily fat macros.

This is why it is vital that you meal plan which is the next big mistake that people make.

2.   Not Meal Planning

This is probably the biggest mistake we see from Keto dieting beginner. The ones that don't meal plan end up falling way short of their daily macros or end up slipping and eating stuff that knocks them out of ketosis because they're hungry.

Yes, meal planning takes a bit of time and preparation but nobody said this was going to be a walk in the park.

Meal planning will not only save you a bunch of headache and frustration, it's a great way to save money as well. When you meal plan, you know exactly what you're going to put into your body on any given day. That means you can make the right adjustments and understand what tweaks you might need to make to your diet.

3.   Too Much Protein

Growing up all you hear is that protein is good for you and it is when it's not consumed in excess. The issue with protein on the ketogenic diet is that because your body is using fats as a fuel source, it only needs proteins to help main muscle mass.

Surprisingly enough, you need much less protein than you'd expect to make this happen. When you consume more protein than your body needs it ends up converting that protein into glucose which, in turn, can raise your blood sugar levels and knock you out of ketosis. Most people have no problem reaching their protein macros because protein seems to be in everything. This is why it's important to meal plan so you understand how much protein you are putting into your body.

4.   Looking For a Quick Fix

It's a shame it's called the ketogenic diet because the reality of the situation is that it's really a lifestyle. You don't do keto for a short period to lose weight and then go back to your old eating habits because then you'll just discover you're back at the very beginning again.

The health benefits of keto show that it's more than worth its time becoming something that you stick with for the rest of your life.

If you're looking for a quick fix then just cut out sugars from your diet. For most people, that will cause a healthy drop in weight without having to meal plan, track your macros, and other things required of you with the keto diet.

5. Not Getting Enough Sleep

Just like water, if you aren't getting the sleep you need your body can't do what it needs to do. It's important that you give your body time to reset so it can tackle another day.

Lack of sleep can also contributes to you slipping up and eating those dozen donuts as you look for quick energy sources.

HOW TO CHECK KETONE LEVELS

Testing ketone levels in your body is the only true way to know whether or not you've entered (and remain in) ketosis. This is important to be sure you're reaping the full benefits of the ketogenic diet here.

When your body starts burning fat for fuel and enters ketosis, the ketones it creates will spill over into your urine, blood, and breath so it's possible to test for them in each area.

Thankfully, there are several methods for testing your ketone levels at home:

Urine testing: You can buy urine strips that indicate your ketone level by color. These can usually be bought at your local drugstore or pharmacy for a low cost.

The downside of urine testing is that they aren't always reliable, especially if you've been in ketosis for a while. When you're more efficient at using ketones, a lower level of ketones might show up even if you're burning through them.

Other factors can affect the reading too, such as hydration and electrolyte levels.

• **Breath Testing:** Acetone is the ketone that shows up on the breath, and you can test it using a breath meter.

After purchasing the breath meter, there are no ongoing costs for testing like with urine strips. However, this method isn't the most reliable and usually should not be your sole method for testing.

• **Blood Testing:** This is the most accurate way to monitor ketone levels. Using a blood glucose meter, you can check ketone levels using a blood strip. Just be warned that this method can be pricey if you test frequently.

For best results, you'll (ideally) be providing your body with optimal nutrition from rich, healthy fat sources, nutritious protein, and other foods that provide the vitamins and minerals the body needs. See our ketogenic diet food list for exactly what to eat to get keto working best for you.

CHAPTER THREE

KETO BAKING TIPS

Best Low Carb Flour

Let's begin this keto baking lesson with choosing the right keto-friendly flours. It's important to note that wheat flour will always be finer and lighter than any alternative low carb flour.

The main reason they don't behave the same is that keto-friendly flours do not have gluten in them. The chewiness that a wheat flour provides will not necessarily translate in a low carb baked good because it lacks gluten.

Keto Flour Alternatives

This is where things can get a bit confusing. There are many low carb choices and it can get overwhelming when you are new to this way of baking.

Each low carb flour alternative acts differently. So, based on what you are trying to convert you will need to choose the one that works best for that particular type of baked good.

Almond flour is the easiest of all the low carb flours to work with. Generally, almond flour is a go-to choice for low-carb cakes, muffin, quick bread, and cookies.

However, the ratio of almond flour called for will depend on the recipe you are making. A cake recipe will not call for the same amount as say a cookie recipe.

Plus, swapping almond flour for wheat flour is not an automatic 1:1 ratio. Why? Because you are dealing with a nut that has been ground. And nuts are high in fat, moisture and void of gluten.

What's more, the texture of wheat flour is much finer and drier than almond flour. This is why good keto baking recipes will consider this.

If that's not enough almond flour weighs much differently from wheat flour. Sometimes, depending on the brand there could be more than an ounce of difference.

You may want to invest in a kitchen scale to ensure you are measuring your ingredients correctly.

Almond Flour Versus Almond Meal

If you've ever attempted to buy almond flour or almond meal you may have noticed a few differences between them.

Almond flour is lighter in color and texture. While almond meal has flecks of brown color in it. This is because an almond meal is made from almonds that have not been peeled.

In the case of almond flour, they are ground much finer and without their skins. The almonds have been blanched to remove their skins before grinding. It's why you do not see any brown specks in the flour.

You may have also noticed that there is a significant price difference between the two. This is because it's more labor-intensive to produce almond flour since they have to go through the blanching process first.

Keep in mind that in addition to their differences, almond flour and meal brands will vary from brand to brand.

You'll notice that some keto baking recipes call for your almond flour to be sifted. Sifting your almond flour will help the texture be finer and will act closer to wheat flour. When I sift my almond flour, I do so after I have measured it.

Note that almond meal will prove to be too heavy and grainy for most of your baked goods.

Coconut Flour

Coconut flour is actually a by-product of coconut milk when it's being produced. Once the coconut milk has been extracted, what's left is coconut meat. The coconut meat is then dried and finely ground. This creates a fine powder that looks a lot like wheat flour.

The biggest difference between wheat flour and that of coconut flour is how dry it is.

Coconut flour needs lots of moisture in the form of liquids and/or eggs in order to be used as a wheat flour alternative. Because coconut flour is quite thirsty it cannot be substituted for flour cup for cup.

Finding the right balance of liquid when using coconut flour can be tricky. If you use too much liquid or eggs you end up with a soggy mess, too little and it won't come together properly.

Just because baking with coconut flour isn't as easy as other low carb flours, it doesn't mean you shouldn't attempt to do so. For those who are allergic to tree nuts, coconut flour can be a great option.

It may require more trial and error when you first start to using coconut flour but when used properly it makes for a great substitute.

Keep in mind that you cannot swap coconut flour 1:1 for almond flour.

The reality is that if you want to swap out almond flour for coconut flour, you will be having to completely change the entire recipe.

Golden Flax Meal

Flax meal is made by simply grinding flaxseeds to produce flour. It can be used well in low carb baking recipes but keep in mind that it's a heavy flour. This is because it's a little more challenging to grind the flaxseeds fine.

Keep in mind that you want to use golden flax meal not regular flax meal in your recipes. Regular flax meal tends to have a gummy texture when baked so it's a no go in my opinion.

Flax eggs are a common substitution for vegan recipes, or for those who are allergic to eggs.

Some people also use flax meal to substitute eggs in a recipe because its texture thickens to a gel-like consistency when water is added.

Keep in mind though that If a recipe is mainly an egg-based recipe, this substitution will probably not work.

To replace 1 egg, mix 1 tablespoon of ground flax meal with 2 1/2 tablespoons of water and allow it to thicken for about 5 minutes. This mixture can be used to replace the eggs but it will not act exactly as eggs do.

Hazelnut Flour

Hazelnut flour is made by grinding hazelnuts. It can be a great substitute for almond flour. Some people prefer this low carb keto flour because it tends to be less grainy and produces a finer product.

It is especially nice in cookie and cake recipes. However, it can be the priciest of all low carb flours since it's not as common.

Sunflower Seed Flour

Sunflower seed flour is produced by grinding sunflower seeds finely, sunflower seeds can be a good low carb flour alternative if you are allergic to nuts. The taste of the sunflowers is pretty pronounced, so it may require using different brands to see which one you like best.

Sunflower seed flour has a great quality in that it can be ground finely. And if you have a great blender, you could even make it at home.

However, does have one negative and it's that it tends to turn a shade of green when baked. This is due to a chemical reaction to baking powder or soda. This doesn't affect the flavor but it may not be as appealing on the eyes.

A tip to avoid this is to add a tablespoon of apple cider vinegar or lemon juice to help counteract this reaction.

Sesame Seed Flour

Created by grinding sesame seeds finely, sesame seed flour is yet another great nut-free option. It is a little harder to come by and may require you make your own by grinding it yourself at home. I've also noticed that not all brands are created equal.

Although, it can be used in place of almond flour, personally, it has a strong taste so I would only recommend using it when you have other flavors to help mask this.

GLUTEN AND STARCH ALTERNATIVES

The gluten in traditional flours gives baked goods structure and it helps bind them together.

Trying to replicate these qualities with flours that have no gluten can sometimes prove to be a challenge.

A solution is to add whey protein, or binders like xanthan gum, psyllium husk, gelatin, cream cheese or extra eggs.

Psyllium

Psyllium is simply pulverized psyllium husk shells and in keto baking, this fiber is used to give more of a bread-like texture to your baked goods, but since it's very high in fiber it is commonly used as a laxative. Having more fiber in our diet is a good thing but if you have a sensitive stomach you need to keep that in mind.

Psyllium is used in keto baking in an attempt to mimic gluten. When it's added to liquid it forms a gel-like substance.

When adding it to a liquid it turns into a gel-like substance. It works a bit like gluten in traditional baking and makes it possible to handle the dough when rolling or shaping it.

Here again, psyllium powders vary greatly from brand to brand. Because another factor with psyllium powder is that some tend to turn purple when baked. Which is not exactly what you are going for.

Xanthan Gum

Xanthan gum is a binding agent. It's what gives your toothpaste its jelly consistency. In keto baking, it's used to take the place of gluten. It's important to note that a little goes a long way with xantham gum. Otherwise you baked goods get a slippery mouth-feel to them.

Whey Protein Isolate Is used commonly in many keto baked goods. Mainly because it helps with the rise.

Gelatin

You may also notice that some low carb baking recipes use gelatin. That's because it helps give baked goods structure and chewiness factor.

Collagen

Adding a few tablespoons of collagen to keto baking can also add a chewy factor similar to gelatin. Although, I recommend you know the brand of collagen since some of them have a pronounced chicken flavor since the majority of products made from collagen use chicken parts.

Baking Powder

When it comes to baking powder and searching for keto-friendly options you will need to check your labels carefully. The reason being that baking powder is just a mixture of three ingredients.

The ingredients are baking soda, cream of tartar, and starch. The inclusion of starch is where some people who need to watch their macros very carefully run into trouble. Because the starch adds carbs to your baked goods.

The problem is that removing the starch and just using baking soda or cream and cream of tartar makes it difficult to measure. The primary role of the starch is to make it easier to measure and as a little bit of a bulking agent.

The number of carbs will vary per brand but in most brands, you are looking at 1 carb per 1/4 teaspoon. In a typical ketogenic baking recipe that can be anywhere from 6 -8 additional carbs for the entire recipe.

That may not seem significant but it can add up rather quickly.

GLUTEN AND STARCH ALTERNATIVES

The gluten in traditional flours gives baked goods structure and it helps bind them together.

Trying to replicate these qualities with flours that have no gluten can sometimes prove to be a challenge.

A solution is to add whey protein, or binders like xanthan gum, psyllium husk, gelatin, cream cheese or extra eggs.

Psyllium

Psyllium is simply pulverized psyllium husk shells and in keto baking, this fiber is used to give more of a bread-like texture to your baked goods but since it's very high in fiber it is commonly used as a laxative. Having more fiber in our diet is a good thing but if you have a sensitive stomach you need to keep that in mind.

Psyllium is used in keto baking in an attempt to mimic gluten. When it's added to liquid it forms a gel-like substance.

When adding it to a liquid it turns into a gel-like substance. It works a bit like gluten in traditional baking and makes it possible to handle the dough when rolling or shaping it.

Here again, psyllium powders vary greatly from brand to brand. Because another factor with psyllium powder is that some tend to turn purple when baked. Which is not exactly what you are going for.

Xanthan Gum

Xanthan gum is a binding agent. It's what gives your toothpaste its jelly consistency. In keto baking, it's used to take the place of gluten. It's important to note that a little goes a long way with xantham gum. Otherwise you baked goods get a slippery mouth-feel to them.

Whey Protein Isolate Is used commonly in many keto baked goods. Mainly because it helps with the rise.

Gelatin

You may also notice that some low carb baking recipes use gelatin. That's because it helps give baked goods structure and chewiness factor.

Collagen

Adding a few tablespoons of collagen to keto baking can also add a chewy factor similar to gelatin. Although, I recommend you know the brand of collagen since some of them have a pronounced chicken flavor since the majority of products made from collagen use chicken parts.

Baking Powder

When it comes to baking powder and searching for keto-friendly options you will need to check your labels carefully. The reason being that baking powder is just a mixture of three ingredients.

The ingredients are baking soda, cream of tartar, and starch. The inclusion of starch is where some people who need to watch their macros very carefully run into trouble. Because the starch adds carbs to your baked goods.

The problem is that removing the starch and just using baking soda or cream and cream of tartar makes it difficult to measure. The primary role of the starch is to make it easier to measure and as a little bit of a bulking agent.

The number of carbs will vary per brand but in most brands, you are looking at 1 carb per 1/4 teaspoon. In a typical ketogenic baking recipe that can be anywhere from 6 -8 additional carbs for the entire recipe.

That may not seem significant but it can add up rather quickly.

CHAPTER FOUR

HEALTHY KETO RECIPES IDEAS

A Ketogenic recipe is a great way to practice healthy eating lifestyle and diet. A low carb dish is not necessarily for those who are on a diet or want to lose their weight. A low carb lifestyle can and should be adopted by all. The advantages of a low carb balanced diet are that it has all the necessary nutrients minus the unhealthy fats. A low carb meal can be had from a choice of almost any kind of dish.

Any dish you wish can be converted into low carb by modifying a few ingredients.

Another essential thing one should realize is there's no such thing as low carb junk food. Junk food is junk food, be it high in carbs or low. It doesn't do much good to your body and your health. So it is wise to reduce or remove junk food entirely from one's meals.

So be knowledgeable about what you eat and be wise. Be healthy!

If you're not sure where to begin have no fear. There are some really delicious, good-for-you keto recipes out there that are begging to be eaten

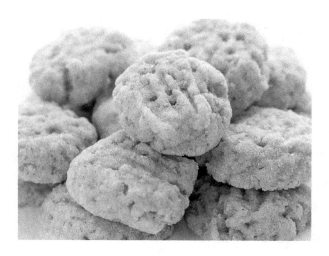

Keto Burger Buns

Ingredients

- 1 cup almond flour
- 2 teaspoons psyllium husk powder
- 1/2 teaspoon baking powder
- 1/2 teaspoon xanthan gum
- 1 teaspoon yeast dried
- 1 teaspoon inulin
- 2 tablespoons warm water
- 1-ounce butter melted
- 3 large eggs room temperature
- 1 teaspoon sesame seeds

Instructions

- In a mixing bowl, add the almond flour, psyllium powder, baking powder, and xanthan gum and mix well.
- Make a well in the center of the dry ingredients and add the yeast and inulin, followed by the warm water. Mix the yeast, inulin, and water and leave to proof for 5 minutes, until the yeast is foamy.
- Add the butter and eggs and mix well.
- Grease a muffin top pan with a little olive oil.
- Even spoon the mixture between 4 holes and sprinkle with the sesame seeds.
- Leave to proof in a warm place for 15 minutes.
- Preheat your oven to 170C/340F.
- Bake the rolls for 15-20 minutes until they are golden brown and spring back when touched.
- Leave to cool on a wire rack before enjoying.

Nutrition

Serving: 90g | Calories: 278kcal | Carbohydrates: 9g | Protein: 12g | Fat: 21g | Saturated Fat: 5g | Cholesterol: 154mg | Sodium: 118mg | Potassium: 159mg | Fiber: 6g | Sugar: 1g | Vitamin A: 380IU | Calcium: 106mg | Iron: 1.9mg

Keto Cheese & Bacon Rolls

Ingredients

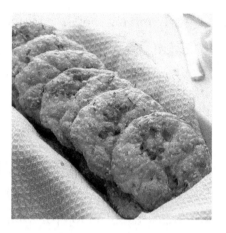

- 5 ounces bacon diced
- 2 tablespoons Cream Cheese
- 2 tablespoons sesame seeds
- 1 tablespoon psyllium husk
- 1 1/2 teaspoons Baking Powder
- 1 cup Cheddar Cheese grated
- 1/2 cup mozzarella cheese grated
- 3 eggs
- 1/2 teaspoon Pepper
- 1 pinch Salt

Instructions

- Preheat oven to 180C/355F.
- Saute diced bacon in a frying pan over medium heat, until just starting to brown. Turn off the heat.
- Add the cream cheese to the bacon and allow to soften while the bacon cools for 5 minutes.
- In your food processor, place the bacon and cream cheese mixture, along with all remaining ingredients. Keep a spoonful of the bacon aside to top the rolls.

- Blend on medium speed for 3-5 minutes until all ingredients are well combined.
- Spoon the mixture into 12 even piles on lined baking dishes. Sprinkle the reserved bacon on each roll.
- Bake for 13-16 minutes until the rolls are golden and puffed up.
- Enjoy them hot from the oven or store in the fridge. They can be quickly reheated in a microwave or toaster oven.

Nutrition

Serving: 1roll | Calories: 149kcal | Carbohydrates: 2g | Protein: 9g | Fat: 12g | Saturated Fat: 7g | Polyunsaturated Fat: 1g | Monounsaturated Fat: 1g | Cholesterol: 3mg | Sodium: 231mg | Potassium: 23mg | Fiber: 2g | Sugar: 0.1g | Vitamin A: 50IU | Calcium: 220mg | Iron: 0.2mg

Low Carb Rosemary & Olive Focaccia Bread

Ingredients

- 4 ounces Cream Cheese softened
- 4 ounces salted butter softened
- 4 large eggs
- 1 3/4 cups almond flour
- 1 teaspoon Baking Powder
- 1/4 teaspoon xanthum gum
- 1/2 teaspoon garlic powder
- 3 sprigs Rosemary
- 16 kalamata olives

Instructions

- Preheat your oven to 190C/375F and line an 8x12in baking pan with parchment paper.
- Place the cream cheese and butter into a mixing bowl and whip using your hand mixers on high speed, until fluffy.
- Add the eggs one at a time and beat well. Don't worry if the mixture looks curdled, it will come together when the dry ingredients are added.
- Add the almond flour, baking powder, xanthum gum, and garlic powder and mix well. Once combined, swap the hand mixer for a spatula and mix well.
- Scoop the mixture onto your prepared baking tray and smooth out.
- Top with the olives and rosemary.
- Place into the oven and bake for 18-25 minutes, the focaccia is cooked when it springs back when touched.
- Enjoy warm or cool and slice to use for sandwiches.

Nutrition

Calories: 284kcal | Carbohydrates: 5g | Protein: 8g | Fat: 26g | Saturated Fat: 10g | Polyunsaturated Fat: 3g | Monounsaturated Fat: 10g | Cholesterol: 114mg | Sodium: 111mg | Potassium: 109mg | Fiber: 2g | Sugar: 1g | Vitamin A: 500IU | Vitamin C: 0.2mg | Calcium: 70mg | Iron: 1.1mg

Keto Soft Pretzels

Ingredients

- 3 cups mozzarella cheese shredded
- 4 tablespoons Cream Cheese
- 1 1/2 cups almond flour
- 2 teaspoons xanthum gum
- 2 eggs room temperature
- 2 teaspoons dried yeast approxiamtely 1 sachet
- 2 tablespoons warm water
- 2 tablespoon butter melted
- 1 tablespoon pretzel salt

Instructions

- Preheat oven to 200C/390F.
- In a microwave-safe dish, place the mozzarella cheese and cream cheese and microwave in 30-sec increments, stirring in between, until fully melted and almost liquid.
- Dissolve the yeast in the warm water and allow it to sit and activate for 2 minutes.
- In your stand mixer (using the dough hook attachment), place the almond meal and xanthum gum and mix well.
- Add the eggs, yeast mixture and 1 tablespoon of the melted butter and mix well.

- Add the hot melted cheese to the stand mixer and allow it to knead the dough until all the ingredients are fully combined. Around 5-10 minutes.
- Split the dough into 12 balls. The dough is easiest to work with while it is warm.
- Roll each ball into a long skinny log and twist into a pretzel shape. Place on a lined cookie sheet and give a little space with side as the pretzels will rise.
- Brush the pretzels with the remaining butter and sprinkle with pretzel salt.
- Bake in the oven for 12-15 minutes.
- When the pretzels are golden brown, remove them from the oven, and don't burn your fingers trying to eat them immediately.

Nutrition

Serving: 1pretzel | Calories: 217kcal | Carbohydrates: 3g | Protein: 11g | Fat: 18g | Saturated Fat: 7g | Polyunsaturated Fat: 2g | Monounsaturated Fat: 7g | Cholesterol: 43mg | Sodium: 615mg | Potassium: 70mg | Fiber: 2g | Sugar: 1g | Vitamin A: 150IU | Calcium: 40mg | Iron: 0.7mg

Gluten-Free Garlic Bread Pretzels with Parmesan Cheese
- Ingredients
- 11 ounces mozzarella cheese shredded

- 4 tablespoons Butter
- 2 teaspoons dried yeast
- 2 tablespoons warm water
- 5.5 ounces almond flour
- 2 teaspoons xanthum gum
- 1 teaspoon garlic powder
- 1/2 teaspoon Salt
- 2 teaspoons dried oregano
- 2 eggs
- 1 tablespoon Butter melted
- 1/3 cup Parmesan cheese finely grated

Instructions

- Preheat oven to 180C/355F.
- In a heatproof bowl, place the mozzarella cheese and 4 tablespoons of butter. Place in the microwave until completely melted & pourable. Or melt in a saucepan on the stove.
- Add the yeast to your mixing bowl and pour over the warm water.
- Add the almond flour, xanthum gum, garlic powder, salt, and oregano. Mix well.
- Add the eggs and lightly mix.
- Add the melted cheese and butter mixture and mix well.

- When to dough is cool enough to handle, put on food-safe disposable gloves and knead until all ingredients are combined.
- Split the mixture into 12 evenly sized balls. Roll each ball into a long sausage and twist into a pretzel shape.
- Place on a cookie sheet lined with parchment paper.
- Once all the pretzels have been rolled, brush them with remaining tablespoon of melted butter and sprinkle over the parmesan cheese.
- Bake in the oven for 15-20 minutes, until the pretzels are golden brown and the edges are firm. Allow to sit for 5 minutes before enjoying!
- Enjoy the pretzels as they are or serve with Roast Garlic Aioli.

Nutrition

Serving: 1pretzel | Calories: 248kcal | Carbohydrates: 3g | Protein: 14g | Fat: 21g | Saturated Fat: 9g | Polyunsaturated Fat: 2g | Monounsaturated Fat: 8g | Cholesterol: 54mg | Sodium: 267mg | Potassium: 89mg | Fiber: 2g | Sugar: 1g | Vitamin A: 250IU | Vitamin C: 0.1mg | Calcium: 120mg | Iron: 0.9mg

Low-Carb Choc Chip

Ingredients

- 3/4 cup coconut flour
- 1 teaspoon Baking Powder
- 2 tablespoons Erythritol

- 6 eggs
- 3/4 cup Sugar-Free Maple Syrup
- 3 ounces Heavy Cream
- 4 ounces butter unsalted, melted
- 3/4 cup Sugar-Free Chocolate Chips
- US Customary - Metric

Instructions

- Preheat oven to 180C/355F
- Place all ingredients, except chocolate chips into your stand mixer. Mix on medium speed for 3 minutes, until all ingredients are combined.
- Allow sitting for 2 minutes to allow the coconut flour to soak up the moisture.
- Mix again on medium for 1 minute, or until there are no lumps.
- Add chocolate chips and combine.
- Spoon mixture into 12 holes of a muffin tin lined with cupcake papers.
- Bake for 20-25 minutes. The muffins are cooked when an inserted skewer comes out clean, and the tops are beginning to brown.
- Place on a wire rack to cool for 10 minutes.

Nutrition

Serving: 1Muffin | Calories: 232kcal | Carbohydrates: 10g | Protein: 3g | Fat: 17g | Saturated Fat: 12g | Polyunsaturated Fat: 0.4g | Monounsaturated Fat: 3g | Cholesterol: 30mg | Sodium: 68mg | Potassium: 8mg | Fiber: 6g | Sugar: 1g | Vitamin A: 350IU | Vitamin C: 0.1mg | Calcium: 10mg | Iron: 2.7mg

Low Carb Savory Cheddar Cheese & Zucchini

Ingredients

- 12 ounces zucchini grated (2 packed cups)
- 1/2 cup Butter melted
- 1/4 teaspoon Salt
- 1/4 teaspoon Pepper
- 6 eggs
- 2 tablespoons oregano finely chopped
- 1 teaspoon Baking Powder
- 3/4 cup coconut flour
- 1 cup Cheddar Cheese grated
- US Customary - Metric

Instructions

- Preheat oven to 180C/355F.
- In a mixing bowl, add the zucchini, butter, salt, and pepper and mix well.
- Add the eggs, oregano and baking powder and mix well.

- Add the coconut flour and mix until the batter becomes thick.

- Fold through the cheddar cheese.

- Line the holes of a standard muffin tin with silicone cupcake molds and evenly divide the mixture between the holes. Overfill each hole creating little piles of soon to be muffins, the muffins don't rise very much.

- Bake for 25 minutes until the muffins are golden.

- Allow cooling for 5 minutes before enjoying.

Nutrition

Serving: 1muffin | Calories: 185kcal | Carbohydrates: 6g | Protein: 7g | Fat: 15g | Saturated Fat: 9g | Polyunsaturated Fat: 1g | Monounsaturated Fat: 3g | Cholesterol: 127mg | Sodium: 165mg | Potassium: 120mg | Fiber: 5g | Sugar: 1g | Vitamin A: 450IU | Vitamin C: 7.4mg | Calcium: 120mg | Iron: 1.6mg

Keto Peanut Butter Cookies

Ingredients

- 12 ounces natural peanut butter crunchy

- 1/2 cup finely shredded coconut unsweetened

- 1/2 cup xylitol

- 2 large eggs

- 1 teaspoon vanilla extract

- US Customary - Metric

Instructions

- Preheat your oven to 160C/320F. Line a cookie sheet with parchment paper and set aside.

- In a mixing bowl, add all ingredients and mix. Be sure to mix all the ingredients thoroughly.

- Roll the mixture into heaped tablespoon-sized balls and press onto your cookie sheet. These cookies do not spread at all so be sure to shape them into your desired size before baking and press with a fork or your fingers to create crunchy ridges. The ridgier (if that's a word), the better.

- Bake in the oven for 12-18 minutes or until the tops of the cookies are browning, and the edges are beginning to harden. They will firm up when cooling but become very dry and sandy if overcooked so be careful.

- Leave cookies to cool completely before enjoying.

Nutrition

Serving: 1cookie | Calories: 111kcal | Carbohydrates: 6g | Protein: 5g | Fat: 7g | Saturated Fat: 2g | Cholesterol: 21mg | Sodium: 100mg | Potassium: 133mg | Fiber: 3g | Sugar: 1g | Vitamin A: 30IU | Calcium: 10mg | Iron: 0.5mg

Keto Shortbread Cookies

Ingredients

- 2 cups almond flour
- 1/3 cup Erythritol
- 1 pinch Salt
- 1 teaspoon vanilla extract
- 1/2 cup Unsalted Butter softened
- 1 large Egg
- US Customary - Metric

Instructions

- Preheat oven to 150C/300F.
- In a mixing bowl, add the almond flour, erythritol, salt and vanilla extract. Mix.
- Add the butter and rub into the dry ingredients until fully combined.
- Add the egg and mix well.
- Take tablespoon-sized pieces of the mixture and roll into balls, then press onto a lined cookie sheet. We recommend using food-safe gloves to stop the mixture from sticking to your hands.
- Leave a gap between the cookies as they will spread slightly.
- Bake for 15-25 minutes until the edges are browned. The cookies will firm up as they cool. If you are using the cookies as

a base for our Jello Chunk Cheesecake, allow them to cook longer so the edges are firm and they are completely browned.

- Leave to cool before storing in an airtight jar, or using as a cheesecake base.

Nutrition

Serving: 1cookie | Calories: 126kcal | Carbohydrates: 2g | Protein: 3g | Fat: 12g | Saturated Fat: 4g | Polyunsaturated Fat: 1g | Monounsaturated Fat: 4g | Cholesterol: 29mg | Sodium: 6mg | Potassium: 48mg | Fiber: 1g | Sugar: 0.4g | Vitamin A: 250IU | Calcium: 30mg | Iron: 0.5mg

The Keto Bread

Ingredients

- 5 tbsp ground psyllium husk powder
- 1¼ cups almond flour
- 2 tsp baking powder
- 1 tsp sea salt
- 1 cup water
- 2 tsp cider vinegar
- 3 egg whites
- 2 tbsp sesame seeds (optional)

Instructions

• Preheat the oven to 350°F (175°C).

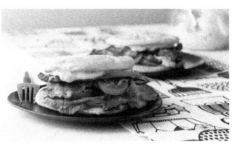

• Mix the dry ingredients in a large bowl. Bring the water to a boil.

• Add vinegar and egg whites to the dry ingredients, and combine well. Add boiling water, while beating with a hand mixer for about 30 seconds. Don't over mix the dough, the consistency should resemble Play-Doh.

• Moisten hands with a little olive oil and shape dough into 6 separate rolls. Place on a greased baking sheet. Top with optional sesame seeds.

• Bake on lower rack in the oven for 50–60 minutes, depending on the size of your bread rolls. They're done when you hear a hollow sound when tapping the bottom of the bun.

• Serve with butter and toppings of your choice.

Keto BLT With Cloud Bread
Ingredients
Cloud bread
• 3 eggs
• 4¼ oz. cream cheese
• 1 pinch salt

- ½ tbsp ground psyllium husk powder
- ½ tsp baking powder
- ¼ tsp cream of tartar (optional)

Toppings
- ½ cup mayonnaise
- 5 oz. bacon
- 2 oz. lettuce
- 1 tomato, thinly sliced
- fresh basil (optional)

Instructions

Cloud bread

• Preheat oven to 300°F (150°C).

• Separate the eggs. Put the egg whites in one bowl and the yolks in another.

• Whip egg whites together with salt (and cream of tartar, if you are using any) until very stiff, preferably using a hand held electric mixer. You should be able to turn the bowl over without the egg whites moving.

• Add cream cheese to the egg yolks and mix well. To make the oopsie more bread-like, add in the optional psyllium seed husk and baking powder.

• Gently fold the egg whites into the egg yolk mixture — try to keep the air in the egg whites.

• Place 8, flattened dough rounds on a parchment paper lined baking tray.

• Bake in the middle of the oven for about 25 minutes, until they turn golden.

Building the BLT

• Fry the bacon in a skillet on medium high heat until crispy.

• Place the cloud bread pieces top-side down.

• Spread 1–2 tablespoon of mayonnaise on each.

• Place lettuce, tomato, some finely chopped fresh basil and fried bacon in layers between the bread halves.

• Serve immediately.

Keto Meat Pie

Ingredients

Pie crust

• ¾ cup almond flour

• 4 tbsp sesame seeds

• 4 tbsp coconut flour

• 1 tbsp ground psyllium husk powder

• 1 tsp baking powder

• 1 pinch salt

• 3 tbsp olive oil or coconut oil, melted

• 1 egg

- 4 tbsp water

Topping

- 8 oz. cottage cheese
- 7 oz. shredded cheese

Filling

- ½ yellow onion, finely chopped
- 1 garlic clove, finely chopped
- 2 tbsp butter or olive oil
- 1¼ lbs ground beef or ground lamb
- 1 tbsp dried oregano or dried basil
- salt and pepper
- 4 tbsp tomato paste or ajvar relish
- ½ cup water

Instructions

1. Preheat the oven to 350°F (175°C).

2. Fry onion and garlic in butter or olive oil over medium heat for a few minutes, until onion is soft. Add ground beef and keep frying. Add oregano or basil. Salt and pepper to taste.

3. Add tomato paste or ajvar relish. Add water. Lower the heat and let simmer for at least 20 minutes. While the meat simmers, make the dough for the crust.

4. Mix all the crust ingredients in a food processor for a few minutes until the dough turns into a ball. If you don't have a food processor, you can mix by hand with a fork.

5. Place a round piece of parchment paper in a well-greased springform pan or deep-dish pie pan — 9-10 inches (23-25 cm) in diameter — to make it easier to remove the pie when it's done. Spread the dough in the pan and up along the sides. Use a spatula or well-greased fingers. Once the crust is shaped to the pan, prick the bottom of the crust with a fork.

6. Pre-bake the crust for 10-15 minutes. Remove from the oven and place the meat in the crust. Mix cottage cheese and shredded cheese together, and layer on top of the pie.

7. Bake on lower rack for 30-40 minutes or until the pie has turned a golden color.

How to vary this recipe

This keto minced meat pie has an easily worked dairy-free pie crust. Here, we have filled it with meat and cheese, but you can use any filling you like. This dish is so versatile, the only limit is your imagination!

If you want a completely dairy-free meal we suggest checking out this keto vegetable pie. Another vegetarian alternative is our very popular keto avocado pie. You can also substitute the meat filling for chicken or salmon.

You can also vary the flavoring of this keto pie. Instead of the dried herbs you can add a couple of tablespoons of Tex-Mex seasoning. Serve it with some leafy greens and avocado, and you'll have the perfect meal for Taco Tuesday.

Feel free to serve this meat pie with a fresh green salad and dressing. Serve lukewarm for peak flavor.

How to store the keto meat pie

Savory pies are perfect for meal prep. Enjoy as much as you want for dinner and then divide any leftovers into portion-sized pieces.

They keep in the fridge for up to 4 days and in the freezer for 2-3 months.

This pie tastes good cold but even better if it's gently reheated in a microwave or in the oven on a low temperature.

Troubleshooting

Nut flours are heat sensitive and should never be baked on high temperatures or they get burnt. If the crust is cooking too fast and is at risk of burning you can prevent that by wrapping aluminium foil on the edge of the crust. This will allow the center to cook and get golden brown, while you keep the edges from burning.

This recipe yields a dough that makes a thin crust. If you have a bigger pie dish or want a thicker crust you can make 1.5 times the recipe for the crust.

Low-Carb Eggplant Pizza

Ingredients

- 2 eggplant
- 1/3 cup olive oil, for brushing and frying
- 2 garlic cloves
- 1 yellow onion
- ¾ lb ground beef
- ¾ cup tomato sauce
- 1 tsp salt
- ½ tsp pepper
- ½ tsp ground cinnamon (optional)
- 10 oz. shredded cheese
- ¼ cup chopped fresh oregano

Instructions

1. Preheat the oven to 400°F (200°C).

2. Slice the eggplants lengthwise, about ⅓–½ inches (1 cm) thick. Coat with olive oil on both sides and place on a baking sheet lined with parchment paper. Bake for about 20 minutes or until slightly browned.

3. Fry garlic and onion in remaining olive oil until softened, about 3-4 minutes.

4. Add beef and sauté until cooked through. Add tomato sauce, and season with salt and pepper. Let simmer for 10 minutes, or until warmed through.

5. Remove the eggplant slices from the oven and spread the meat mixture on top. Sprinkle with cheese and oregano. Place in the oven for about 10 minutes or until the cheese has melted.

6. Serve with a green salad dressed with olive oil.

Low-Carb Sloppy Joe's

Ingredients

The bread

- 1¼ cups almond flour
- 5 tbsp ground psyllium husk powder
- 2 tsp baking powder
- 1 tsp sea salt
- 2 tsp cider vinegar
- 1¼ cups boiling water
- 3 egg whites
- sesame seeds (optional)

Meat sauce

- 2 tbsp olive oil
- 1 yellow onion
- 4 garlic cloves
- 1½ lbs ground beef
- 4 tbsp tomato paste
- 14 oz. crushed tomatoes
- 1 tbsp chili powder

- 1 tbsp Dijon mustard
- 1 tbsp red wine vinegar
- 2 tsp salt
- ¼ tsp ground black pepper

Toppings

- ½ cup mayonnaise
- 6 oz. shredded cheese

Instructions

The bread

1. Preheat the oven to 350°F (175°C). Mix the dry ingredients in a bowl.

2. Add the vinegar, boiling water, and egg whites to the bowl. Whisk the dough with a hand mixer for about 30 seconds. Don't overmix it. (You want the consistency to resemble Play-Doh.)

3. With moistened hands, form the dough into 4 or 8 pieces of bread.

4. Bake on lower rack in oven for 50–60 minutes, depending on the size of your bread. They're done when you hear a hollow sound when tapping the bottom of the bun.

Meat sauce

1. Sauté onion and garlic in a large frying pan over medium-high until the onion is soft and translucent.

2. Add the ground beef to the pan and increase the heat a little. Fry the meat thoroughly.

3. Add the other ingredients and mix well.

4. Let simmer for at least 15 minutes on low heat until most of the liquid is reduced.

5. Taste and add more seasoning if needed.

6. Serve in low-carb bread with a lot of shredded cheese and a dollop of mayonnaise.

Tip!

Embrace your creativity! Sprinkle poppy or sesame seeds on the bread before baking. Or why not some salt flakes and herbs? You can also make hot dog or hamburger buns out of the dough.

Six pieces of this bread contain about 2 grams of carbs per bun.

Save those leftovers! The meat sauce can be kept in the fridge for up to three days, or in the freezer. And don't get stuck in a rut. Feel free to use any kind of meat you want – beef, lamb, poultry or pork.

Keto Tortilla With Ground Beef And Salsa

Ingredients

Low-carb tortillas

• 2 eggs

• 2 egg whites

• 5 oz. cream cheese softened

• ½ tsp salt

• 1½ tsp ground psyllium husk powder

• 1 tbsp coconut flour

Filling

- 2 tbsp olive oil
- 1 lb ground beef or ground lamb, at room temperature
- 2 tbsp Tex-Mex seasoning
- ½ cup water
- salt and pepper

Salsa

- 2 avocados, diced
- 1 tomato, diced
- 2 tbsp lime juice
- 1 tbsp olive oil
- ½ cup fresh cilantro, chopped
- salt and pepper

For serving

- 6 oz. shredded Mexican cheese
- 3 oz. shredded lettuce

Instructions

Low-carb tortillas

1. Preheat the oven to 400°F (200°C).

2. Using an electric mixer with the whisk attachment, whisk the eggs and egg whites until fluffy, preferably for a few minutes. In a separate large bowl, beat the cream cheese until smooth. Add the eggs to the cream cheese, and whisk until the eggs and cream cheese form a smooth batter.

3. Mix salt, psyllium husk and coconut flour in a small bowl. Add the flour mix one spoon at a time into the batter and continue to whisk some more. Let the batter sit for a few minutes or until the batter is thick like an American pancake batter. How fast the batter will swell depends on the brand of psyllium husk – some trial and error might be needed.

4. Bring out two baking sheets and place parchment paper on each. Using a spatula, spread the batter thinly (no more than ¼ inch thick) into 4–6 circles or 2 rectangles.

5. Bake on upper rack for about 5 minutes or more, until the tortilla turns a little brown around the edges. Carefully check the bottom side so that it doesn't burn.

Filling

1. Place a large frying pan over medium-high heat and heat up the oil. Add the ground beef and fry until cooked through.

2. Add the tex-mex seasoning and water and stir. Let simmer until most of the water is gone. Taste to see if it needs additional seasoning.

Salsa and serving

1. Make the salsa from avocado, tomatoes, lime juice, olive oil and fresh cilantro. Salt and pepper to taste.

2. Serve beef filling in a tortilla, with shredded cheese, salsa and shredded leafy greens.

Tip!

Bring the ground beef out of the refrigerator a while before frying. Cold ground beef will cool down the frying pan and the ground beef will be boiled and not fried. The latter tastes a lot better.

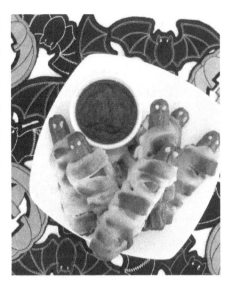

Keto Mummy Dogs

Ingredients

- ½ cup almond flour
- 4 tbsp coconut flour
- ½ tsp salt
- 1 tsp baking powder
- 2½ oz. butter
- 6 oz. shredded cheese
- 1 egg
- 1 lb sausages in links, or uncured hot dogs
- 1 egg, for brushing the dough
- 16 cloves, for the mummies eyes (optional)

Instructions

1. Preheat the oven to 350°F (175°C).

2. Mix almond flour, coconut flour and baking powder in a large bowl.

3. Melt the butter and cheese in a pan on low heat. Stir thoroughly with a wooden spoon, for a smooth and flexible batter. After a few minutes, remove from heat.

4. Stir the egg into to the flour mixture, and then add the cheese mixture, combining all until it becomes a firm dough.

5. Flatten into a rectangle, about 8×14 inches (20×35 cm).

6. Cut into 8 long strips, less than an inch wide (1.5–2 cm).

7. Wrap the dough strips around the hot dog and brush with a whisked egg.

8. Place on a baking sheet lined with parchment paper and bake for 15–20 minutes until the dough is golden brown. The hot dog will be done by then too.

9. Push two cloves into each hot dog to make them look like eyes – but only for decoration. Don't eat the cloves!

Tip!

Using larger hot dogs? Pre-fry them for a couple of minutes before wrapping them up in the cheese dough and baking.

Low-Carb Tortilla Pizza

Ingredients

Topping

- ½ cup unsweetened tomato sauce
- 8 oz. shredded cheese
- 2 tsp dried basil or dried oregano
- salt and pepper (optional)

Low-carb tortillas

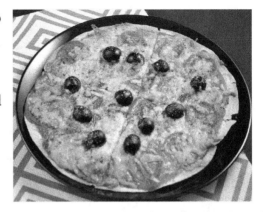

- 2 eggs
- 2 egg whites
- 6 oz. cream cheese
- ¼ tsp salt
- 1 tsp ground psyllium husk powder
- 1 tbsp coconut flour

Instructions

Tortillas

1. Preheat the oven to 400°F (200°C).

2. Whisk the eggs and egg whites fluffy and continue to whisk with a hand mixer, preferably for a few minutes. Add cream cheese and continue to whisk until the batter is smooth.

3. Mix salt, psyllium husk and coconut flour in a small bowl. Add the flour mix one spoon at a time into the batter and continue to

whisk some more. Let the batter sit for a few minutes, or until the batter is thick like an American pancake batter. How fast the batter will swell depends on the brand of psyllium husk – some trial and error might be needed.

4. Bring out two baking sheets and place parchment paper on each. Using a spatula, spread the batter thinly (no more than ¼ inch thick) into 4–6 circles or 2 rectangles.

5. Bake on upper rack for about 5 minutes or more, until the tortilla turns a little brown around the edges. Carefully check the bottom side so that it doesn't burn.

Pizza

1. Turn your oven up to 450°F (225°C).

2. Spread 1-2 tablespoons of tomato paste, sauce or ajvar (roasted red pepper sauce) on each low-carb tortilla bread. Salt and pepper if needed.

3. Bake the mini pizzas in the oven until the cheese has melted.

Tip!

These little guys made from low-carb tortilla bread are perfect as a snack or appetizer. If you'd love to make a meal for the whole family, follow this recipe for a low-carb pizza.

Keto Tuna Cheese Melt

Ingredients

Oopsie bread

- 3 eggs
- 4½ oz. cream cheese
- 1 pinch salt
- ½ tbsp ground psyllium husk powder
- ½ tsp baking powder

Tuna mix

- 1 cup mayonnaise or sour cream
- 4 celery stalks
- ½ cup dill pickles, chopped
- 8 oz. tuna in olive oil
- 1 tsp lemon juice
- 1 garlic clove, minced
- salt and pepper, to taste

Topping

- 2/3 lb shredded cheese
- ¼ tsp cayenne pepper or paprika powder

For serving

- 5 oz. leafy greens
- olive oil

Instructions

Oopsie bread

1. Preheat the oven to 300°F (150°C).

2. Separate the egg yolks into one bowl and the egg whites into another.

3. Whip egg whites together with salt until very stiff. You should be able to turn the bowl over without the egg whites moving.

4. Mix the egg yolks and the cream cheese well. Add the psyllium seed husk and baking powder.

5. Gently fold the egg whites into the egg yolk mix – try to keep the air in the egg whites.

6. Make 2 oopsies per serving and place on a parchment-lined baking tray.

7. Bake in the middle of the oven for about 25 minutes – until they turn golden.

Tuna mix and serving

1. Preheat the oven to 350°F (175°C).

2. Mix the salad ingredients well.

3. Place the bread slices on a baking sheet lined with parchment paper. Spread the tuna mix on the bread and sprinkle cheese on top.

4. Add some paprika powder or cayenne pepper.

5. Bake in oven until the cheese has turned a nice color, about 15 minutes. Serve the sandwich with some leafy greens drizzled with olive oil.

Low-carb banana waffles

Ingredients

- 1 ripe banana
- 4 eggs
- ¾ cup almond flour
- ¾ cup coconut milk
- 1 tbsp ground psyllium husk powder
- 1 pinch salt
- 1 tsp baking powder
- ½ tsp vanilla extract
- 1 tsp ground cinnamon
- coconut oil or butter, for frying

Instructions

1. Mix all of the ingredients together and let sit for a while.

2. Make in a waffle maker or fry in a frying pan with coconut oil or butter.

3. Serve with hazelnut spread or whipped coconut cream and some fresh berries, or just have them as is with melted butter. You can't go wrong!

Tip!

Got extra ripe bananas? Make more waffles and freeze the leftovers for a quick and easy future morning. Wrap each pancake individually in plastic wrap for easy defrosting.

Here's how to whip coconut cream. Let a can of coconut milk sit in the refrigerator for at least 4 hours to separate the cream from the water. Open the can carefully and remove the cream part with a spoon. Place in a bowl and whisk with a hand blender for a few minutes.

Keto Pancakes With Berries And Whipped Cream

Ingredients

Pancakes

- 4 eggs
- 7 oz. cottage cheese
- 1 tbsp ground psyllium husk powder
- 2 oz. butter or coconut oil

Toppings

- 2 oz. fresh raspberries or fresh blueberries or fresh strawberries
- 1 cup heavy whipping cream

Instructions

1. Add eggs, cottage cheese and psyllium husk to a medium size bowl and mix together. Let sit for 5-10 minutes to thicken up a bit.

2. Heat up butter or oil in a non-stick skillet. Fry the pancakes on medium-low heat for 3–4 minutes on each side. Don't make them too big or they will be hard to flip.

3. Add cream to a separate bowl and whip until soft peaks form.

4. Serve the pancakes with the whipped cream and berries of your choice.

Low-Carb Pumpkin Pie

Ingredients

Pie crust

• 3 oz. butter, at room temperature

• ¾ cup coconut flour

• 6 tbsp hazelnut flour

• ¼ tsp ground cinnamon

• ¼ tsp vanilla extract

Pumpkin filling

• ¾ lb pumpkins peeled and diced

• 2 oz. butter

• 1 cup heavy whipping cream

• 2 eggs

• 2 tsp pumpkin pie spice

• 1 pinch salt

Topping

• 1½ cups heavy whipping cream

• ½ lemon, only the zest

Instructions

1. Preheat the oven to 350°F (175°).

2. Put the ingredients for the pie crust in a bowl and mix together into a firm dough.

3. Divide the dough into eight small forms, 3 inches (8 cm) in diameter, or one larger springform.

4. Prebake for 10 minutes if you're making small pies and 15 minutes for one large pie.

5. Meanwhile, make the filling. Put the pumpkin cubes in a pan together with heavy cream and butter.

6. Bring to a boil, reduce heat, and let simmer on medium low until the pumpkin is soft and most of the cream is absorbed. It will take at least 15–20 minutes. Keep stirring. Set aside and let cool a little.

7. Add eggs and spices and mix into a smooth puree with a hand blender or in a food processor.

8. Pour the filling into the pie crust and bake for 15–20 minutes until the filling is firm, a little longer for a large form.

9. It may be a good idea to lower the heat towards the end and cover the edges with a strip of aluminum foil so that the crust doesn't burn.

10. Whisk the heavy cream with a hand mixer until soft peaks form and stir in the lemon zest. Serve with the pie.

Tip!

If you're limiting your dairy intake, you can replace the heavy cream with a creamy coconut milk. For the crust and filling you can replace butter with coconut oil or ghee. The pie freezes well, which means if you make a couple of extra pies you'll always have one ready for unexpected company!

Crustless Low-Carb Pumpkin Pie

Ingredients

- 2 tbsp butter, for greasing the baking dish
- 4 tbsp unsweetened shredded coconut
- 1 lb pumpkins
- 2/3 cup heavy whipping cream
- 1 oz. butter
- ¼ tsp salt
- 2 tsp pumpkin pie spice
- 2 tbsp coconut flour (optional)
- ¼ lemon, only the zest
- 1 tsp baking powder
- 3 eggs
- 1½ cups heavy whipping cream, for serving

Instructions

1. Dice the pumpkin into cubes and place in a pan. Add whipping cream, butter and salt and bring to a boil over medium heat.

2. Lower the heat, let simmer until the pumpkin is soft. It will take at least 15–20 minutes. Stir occasionally.

3. When the pumpkin is soft, add the remaining ingredients, except for the eggs, and blend to a smooth purée using a hand mixer, immersion blender or food processor.

4. Beat the eggs in a separate bowl with a hand mixer for 2–3 minutes. Add the puréed pumpkin and mix well.

5. Preheat the oven to 400°F (200°C). Grease a 9" baking dish with butter and apply the coconut flakes evenly.

6. Pour the batter into the baking dish and bake for about 20 minutes or until set in the middle.

7. Serve with a dollop of whipped heavy cream.

Tip!

The pie will taste its best if you use fresh pumpkin instead of readymade pumpkin purée which contains less carbohydrates, but won't give the pie its natural sweetness. You want all the pumpkin goodness in this fantastic pie

Low-Carb Chocolate And Peanut Squares

Ingredients

• 3½ oz. dark chocolate with a minimum of 70% cocoa solids

• 4 tbsp butter or coconut oil

• 1 pinch salt

• ¼ cup peanut butter

• ½ tsp vanilla extract

• 1 tsp licorice powder or ground cinnamon or ground cardamom (green)

• 1½ oz. salted peanuts, finely chopped or hazelnuts

Instructions

1. Melt chocolate and butter or coconut oil in the microwave oven or in a double boiler. If you don't have a double boiler you can put a

glass bowl on top of a pot of steaming water. Make sure that the water doesn't reach the bowl. The chocolate will melt from the heat of the steam. Set the melted chocolate aside to cool for a few minute before proceeding with the next step.

2. Add all remaining ingredients except the nuts and blend until incorporated.

3. Pour the batter into a small greased baking dish lined with parchment paper (no bigger than 4x6 inches).

4. Top with finely chopped peanuts. Place in the refrigerator to chill.

5. When the batter is set, cut into small squares with a sharp knife. Remember, keep these and all treats small — no more than a 1x1 inch square. Store in the refrigerator or freezer.

Tip

Almond or hazelnut butter work, too. And try different toppings: toasted (and coarsely chopped) almonds or hazelnuts, roasted sesame seeds with unsweetened coconut flakes, or even tahini. Mmmmm…

Low-Carb Chocolate Cake

Ingredients

- 1 tbsp butter or coconut oil, for greasing the pan
- 9 oz. dark chocolate with a minimum of 70% cocoa solids
- 5 oz. butter
- 5 eggs

- 1 pinch salt
- 1 tsp vanilla extract

Instructions

1. Preheat the oven to 320°F (160°C). Use a springform pan, maximum 9 inches (20-22 cm) in diameter. Grease the form with butter or coconut oil and fasten a piece of round parchment paper to the bottom.

2. Break the chocolate into pieces and dice the butter. Melt together using a double boiler or the microwave oven. Be careful — chocolate burns easily so stir often. Once melted, stir until smooth and let the mix cool just a little.

3. Separate the eggs and put the yolks and whites in separate bowls. Add salt to the egg whites and beat with a mixer until stiff peaks form. Set aside.

4. Add vanilla to the egg yolks and whisk until smooth.

5. Pour the melted chocolate and butter into the egg yolks and mix well. Fold in the egg whites. Keep folding just until you can't see any white streaks from the egg whites.

6. Pour the batter into the springform pan and bake for about 15 minutes. To test for doneness, insert a toothpick; it should come out with moist crumbs, not runny batter.

Tip!

Serve at room temperature or even a little warmer. And don't forget a little whipped heavy cream (sour cream is delicious, too) and a few berries if you like!

Low-Carb Coconut Pancakes

Ingredients

- 6 eggs
- 1 pinch salt
- 2 tbsp melted coconut oil
- ¾ cup coconut milk
- ½ cup coconut flour
- 1 tsp baking powder
- butter or coconut oil, for frying

Instructions

1. Separate the yolks from the egg whites and whip the egg whites and pinch of salt with a hand mixer. Continue whipping until stiff peaks form and then set aside.

2. In a separate bowl, whisk together yolks, oil and coconut milk.

3. Add coconut flour and baking powder. Mix into a smooth batter.

4. Gently fold the egg whites into the batter. Let batter rest for 5 minutes.

5. Fry in butter or coconut oil for a couple of minutes or so on each side on low to medium heat. Flip carefully!

6. Serve with melted butter and/or fresh berries.

Low-Carb Granola Bars

Ingredients

- 3 oz. almonds
- 3 oz. walnuts
- 2 oz. sesame seeds
- 2 oz. pumpkin seeds
- 1 oz. flaxseed
- 2 oz. unsweetened shredded coconut
- 2 oz. dark chocolate with a minimum of 70% cocoa solids
- 6 tbsp coconut oil
- 4 tbsp tahini (sesame paste)
- 1 tsp vanilla extract
- 2 tsp ground cinnamon
- 1 pinch sea salt
- 2 eggs
- 3 oz. dark chocolate with a minimum of 70% cocoa solids, for garnish (optional)

Instructions

1. Preheat the oven to 350°F (175°C).
2. Mix all the ingredients in a blender or food processor until they are coarsely chopped.

3. Spoon the mixture into a 7x11 baking dish, preferably lined with parchment paper.

4. Bake for 15–20 minutes, or until the cake has turned golden brown.

5. Let cool a little and remove from the baking dish. Divide into 20 or 24 pieces with a sharp knife.

6. Melt the chocolate in a water bath using a double boiler or in the micro-wave oven.

7. Dip each bar in the chocolate, but just about half an inch or on just one side. Let cool completely.

8. Keep in the refrigerator or freezer.

Tip!

Just use your favorite nuts and seeds, or what you have on hand. A healthy nut and seed mix could consist of equal parts of almonds/hazel nuts/macadamia nuts, pecan nuts/walnuts, sunflower seeds, pumpkin seeds, sesame seeds and flax seeds.

The tahini (sesame paste) can be substituted with almond or nut butter. But remember that for example, peanut butter has a lot more carbohydrates than sesame paste. Let your imagination run wild!

Low-Carb Baked Apples

Ingredients

• 2 oz. butter, at room temperature

• 1 oz. pecans or walnuts

- 4 tbsp coconut flour
- ½ tsp ground cinnamon
- ¼ tsp vanilla extract
- 1 tart/sour apple

For serving

- ¾ cup heavy whipping cream
- ½ tsp vanilla extract

Instructions

1. Preheat the oven to 350°F (175°C). Mix soft butter, chopped nuts, coconut flour, cinnamon and vanilla into a crumbly dough.

2. Rinse the apple, but don't peel it or remove the seeds. Cut off both ends and cut the middle part in four slices.

3. Place the slices in a greased baking dish and add dough crumbs on top. Bake for 15 minutes or more or until the crumbs turn golden brown.

4. Add heavy whipping cream and vanilla to a medium-sized bowl and whip until soft peaks form.

5. Let the apples cool for a couple of minutes and serve with a dollop of whipped cream.

No Bake Keto Peanut Butter Chocolate Bars
Ingredients
For the Bars

- 3/4 cup Almond Flour
- 2 oz Butter
- 1/4 cup Swerve Icing sugar style
- 1/2 cup Creamy Peanut Butter
- Vanilla extract

For the Topping
- 1/2 cup Sugar-Free Chocolate Chips

Instructions

1. Mix all the ingredients for the bars together and spread into a small 6 inch pan

2. Melt the chocolate chips in a microwave oven for 30 seconds and stir.

3. Add another 10 seconds if needed to melt fully.

4. Spread the topping on top of the bars.

5. Refrigerate for at least an hour or two until the bars thicken up. These bars definitely improve with keeping so don't be in a huge rush to eat them

Keto Almond Shortbread

Ingredients
- 1/2 cup Butter
- 1/2 cup Truvia
- 1 teaspoon Almond Extract

• 1 cup Almond Flour

Instructions

1. Preheat the oven to 350F. Lightly grease a 6-inch round baking pan and set it aside.

2. Using a stand mixer, blend together the butter and Truvia, about 3-4 minutes.

3. Add 1 teaspoon almond extract and blend, 30 seconds.

4. Add almond flour little by little and blend, another 2 minutes.

5. Remove the dough and pat it into the baking tin.

6. Bake for 15-20 minutes.

7. Remove the pan carefully and while the shortbread is still warm and soft, cut into 8 pie shaped pieces.

8. Allow the shortbread to cool before serving.

Notes

• You can substitute lemon extract and a little lemon zest for the almond extract.

Nutrition

Calories: 182kcal | Carbohydrates: 3g | Protein: 3g | Fat: 18g | Saturated Fat: 7g | Fiber: 1g

Keto Pie Crust

Ingredients

- 1 cup Almond Flour
- 2 tablespoons Powdered Swerve
- 1/4 cup Melted Coconut Oil

Instructions

1. In a small bowl, mix together almond flour and powdered Swerve.

2. Pour in the melted coconut butter and mix well until you have a crumbly mixture.

3. Tip the mixture into a 9-inch shallow pie pan. Use your fingers to pat the pie crust evenly into the bottom and then work your way up the sides.

4. Once the mixture is evenly spread through the pan, use the tines of a fork to prick the bottom of the crust.

5. Bake at 400F for 8-10 minutes. If you find the top starting to brown faster than the rest, either cover the edges with foil, or reduce the temperature to 375F.

6. Allow the crust to cool for 30 minutes and then fill with the filling of your choice. The French Silk Pudding would be perfect for this crust.

Nutrition

Calories: 137kcal | Carbohydrates: 6g | Protein: 2g | Fat: 13g | Saturated Fat: 6g | Fiber: 1g

Gluten-Free Spiced Keto Cookies

Ingredients

Cream Together

• 4 tbsp softened butter or coconut oil

• 2 tbsp agave nectar (or sub water if your macros can't take it)

• 1 egg

• 2 tablespoons water

Add Dry Ingredients

• 2.5 cup Almond Flour

• 1/3 cup Truvia or 1/2 cup sugar

• 2 tsp ground ginger

• 1 tsp ground cinnamon

• ½ tsp Ground Nutmeg

• 1 tsp Baking Soda

• ¼ tsp Salt

Instructions

1. Preheat the oven to 350F.

2. Line a cookie sheet with parchment paper and set aside.

3. Using a hand blender, cream together the butter, agave nectar, egg, and water.

4. To this mixture, add all the dry ingredients and mix well on low speed.

5. Roll into 2 tsp balls and arrange on a baking tray with parchment paper. They don't really spread too much but leave a little room between them.

6. Bake for 12-15 mins until the tops have lightly browned.

7. Once cooled, store in an air-tight container. For like, the one hour these will be around before you eat them all.

Nutrition

Calories: 122kcal | Carbohydrates: 5g | Protein: 3g | Fat: 10g | Saturated Fat: 2g | Fiber: 1g | Sugar: 2g

Low Carb Chocolate Chip Cookies

Ingredients

- 1.5 cups Almond Flour
- 1 teaspoon Baking Powder
- 1/2 teaspoon Salt
- 1/2 cup Butter
- 1/2 cup Truvia
- 1 teaspoon vanilla extract
- 1 large egg

- 1 cup Sugar-Free Chocolate Chips
- 1/2 cup chopped nuts

Instructions

1. In a stand mixer with a paddle attachment, cream together butter and Truvia.

2. Add egg and mix.

3. Add almond flour, baking powder, salt, and vanilla extract and mix well.

4. Fold in chocolate chips, and nuts.

5. Drop by heaped tablespoons onto a greased baking sheet to make 24 cookies.

6. Bake at 350F for 14-15 minutes until done.

Nutrition

Calories: 120kcal | Carbohydrates: 3g | Protein: 2g | Fat: 11g | Saturated Fat: 4g | Fiber: 1g

Pressure Cooker Keto Almond Carrot Cake

Ingredients

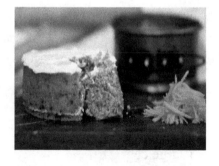

- 3 eggs
- 1 cup Almond Flour
- 2/3 cup Swerve
- 1 teaspoon Baking Powder
- 1.5 teaspoons Apple Pie Spice

- 1/4 cup Coconut Oil
- 1/2 cup Heavy Whipping Cream
- 1 cup carrots shredded
- 1/2 cup walnuts chopped

Instructions

1. Grease a 6-inch cake pan.

2. Mix together all ingredients using a hand mixer, until the mixture is well-incorporated, and looks fluffy. This will keep the cake from being dense as almond flour cakes can sometimes be.

3. Pour into the greased pan and cover the pan with foil.

4. In the inner liner of your Instant Pot, place two cups of water, and a steamer rack. Place the foil-covered cake on the trivet.

5. Press the CAKE button and allow it to cook for 40 minutes. Allow the pressure to release naturally for 10 minutes. Release remaining pressure. If you don't have a cake button, just set your pressure cooker for 40 minutes at high pressure.

6. Let it cool before icing with a frosting of your choice or serve plain.

Nutrition

Calories: 268kcal | Carbohydrates: 6g | Protein: 6g | Fat: 25g | Saturated Fat: 10g | Fiber: 2g | Sugar: 1g

Cream Cheese Pound Cake

Instructions

1. Preheat oven to 350 degrees. Grease a 6-cup bundt pan and set aside. In a large stand-up mixer bowl using the paddle attachment on the mixer, beat together the butter, cream cheese, and Swerve until light and fluffy and well incorporated.

2. Add the almond extract and mix well.

3. Add the eggs and sour cream and mix well.

4. Add all the dry ingredients until well combined. Beat the mixture until it is light and fluffy.

5. Pour the batter into the greased bundt pan. Bake for 40 minutes until a toothpick inserted to the bottom of it comes clean.

Notes

• For an easy sweet tooth fix, cut up slices and freeze individual slices

• You MUST use almond flour for this recipe

• Beat the batter well!

• Use a Six cup bundt pan, not the large 10-12 cup pan

Nutrition

Calories: 304kcal | Carbohydrates: 7g | Protein: 9g | Fat: 27g | Saturated Fat: 8g | Fiber: 2g | Sugar: 1g

Keto Chocolate Cake

Ingredients

- 1 cup Almond Flour
- 2/3 cup Swerve
- 1/4 cup Unsweetened Cocoa Powder
- 1/4 cup chopped walnuts
- 1 teaspoon Baking Powder
- 3 eggs
- 1/3 cup Heavy Whipping Cream
- 1/4 cup Coconut Oil

Instructions

For the Oven

1. Grease an 8-inch cake pan. Turn oven to 350F

2. Mix together all ingredients using a hand mixer, until the mixture is well-incorporated, and looks fluffy. This will keep the cake from being dense as almond flour cakes can sometimes be.

3. Pour into the greased pan and bake for 25-30 minutes until a knife inserted in the center emerges clean.

For the Instant Pot

1. Mix together all ingredients using a hand mixer, until the mixture is well-incorporated, and looks fluffy. This will keep the cake from being dense as almond flour cakes can sometimes be.

2. Grease a heat-proof pan that fits inside your Instant Pot or Pressure Cooker. Pour the cake batter into this pan. I used a 3-cup Bundt Pan

3. In the inner liner of your Instant Pot, place two cups of water, and a steamer rack. Place the foil-covered pot on the trivet.

4. Close the Instant Pot, and cook for 20 minutes under high pressure, and allow the pressure to release naturally for 10 minutes. Release remaining pressure.

Notes

• Make sure to beat the batter very well so your cake is not heavy.

• The cake is sweet enough on its own, but you can use whipped cream for a additional indulgence. Or top with my Two-Ingredient Icing.

• Use a metal pan, but if you only have a glass one be sure it's oven proof. Glass doesn't conduct heat as well as Metal does, so you may have to cook it longer.

Nutrition

Calories: 301kcal | Carbohydrates: 7g | Protein: 8g | Fat: 28g | Saturated Fat: 12g | Cholesterol: 99mg | Sodium: 37mg | Potassium: 183mg | Fiber: 3g | Vitamin A: 315IU | Calcium: 98mg | Iron: 1.8mg

Keto Flourless Chocolate Brownies

Ingredients

- 1/2 cup Sugar-Free Chocolate Chips
- 1/2 cup Butter
- 3 eggs
- 1/4 cup Truvia or other sweetener
- 1 tsp Vanilla extract

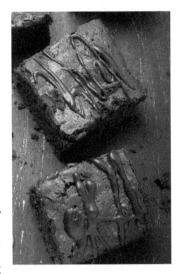

Instructions

1. In a microwave safe bowl, melt butter and chocolate for about 1 minute. Remove and stir well. You really want to use the heat within the butter and chocolate to melt the rest of the clumps. If you microwave until it's all melted, you've overcooked the chocolate. So get a spoon and start stirring. Add 10 seconds if needed but stir well before you decide to do that.

2. In a bowl, add eggs, sweetener, and vanilla and blend until light and frothy.

3. Pour the melted butter and chocolate into the bowl in a slow stream and beat again until it is well-incorporated.

4. Pour the mixture into greased springform container or cake pan and bake at 350F for 30-35 minutes until a knife inserted in the center emerges clean.

5. Serve with whipped cream if desired (see note)

Nutrition

Calories: 224kcal | Carbohydrates: 3g | Protein: 4g | Fat: 23g | Saturated Fat: 13g | Cholesterol: 122mg | Sodium: 169mg | Potassium: 121mg | Fiber: 1g | Vitamin A: 590IU | Calcium: 28mg | Iron: 2.3mg

Lemon Poppy Seed Muffins with Ricotta

Ingredients

- 1 cup Almond Flour
- 1/3 cup Swerve or alternative sweetener
- 1 teaspoon Baking Powder
- 1/4 cup full fat ricotta cheese
- 1/4 cup Coconut Oil
- 3 eggs
- 2 tablespoons Poppy Seeds,
- 4 True lemon packets
- 1/4 cup Heavy Whipping Cream
- 1 teaspoon Lemon Extract

Instructions

1. Mix together all ingredients and beat well until fluffy.

2. Line a muffin pan with silicone cupcake liners.

3. Pour the batter into a muffin pan, dividing equally into 12 servings.

4. Bake at 350F for 40 minutes or until a knife inserted into the center emerges clean.

5. Cool slightly before removing from liners.

Notes

1. You can check whether they're done baking by inserting either a toothpick or a knife into the center of the muffin. If it comes out clean, they're done.

2. I used silicone cupcake liners so they'd pop out easily, but I suspect they might have anyway. However, I always err on the side of caution when baking, as no one wants their baked goods falling apart when taking them out of the pan!

3. Though I used True Lemon packets in this recipe, I think lemon juice and lemon zest would do equally well. Feel free to experiment with it and let me know how it came out in the comments!

4. Though this recipe is for Lemon Poppy Seed Muffins, you can use other flavors such as orange extract or almond to make the same basic recipe 100 different ways. The possibilities are limitless!

Nutrition

Calories: 141kcal | Carbohydrates: 2g | Protein: 4g | Fat: 13g | Saturated Fat: 6g | Cholesterol: 50mg | Sodium: 22mg | Potassium: 68mg | Fiber: 1g | Vitamin A: 155IU | Calcium: 76mg | Iron: 0.7mg

Keto Low Carb Chocolate Peanut Butter Hearts

Ingredients

- 2 cups smooth peanut butter Can use any nut or seed butter
- 3/4 cup sticky sweetener of choice * See notes
- 1 cup coconut flour
- 1-2 cups chocolate chips of choice

Instructions

1. Line a large plate or tray with parchment paper and set aside.

2. In a microwave-safe bowl or stovetop, combine your peanut butter with sticky sweetener and melt until combined.

3. Add your coconut flour and mix well. If the batter is too thin, add more coconut flour. Allow sitting for 10 minutes, to thicken.

4. Form 18-20 small balls of peanut butter dough. Press each ball in a heart-shaped cookie cutter, and remove excess peanut butter dough from the edges. Place peanut butter hearts on the lined plate and refrigerate.

5. Melt your chocolate chips of choice. Using two forks, dip each peanut butter heart in the chocolate until evenly coated. Once all the peanut butter hearts are covered in chocolate, refrigerate until firm.

Notes

* See the post for alternatives to this sticky sweetener.

Keto Low Carb Chocolate Peanut Butter Hearts (Vegan) can keep at room temperature, in a sealed container for up to 2 weeks. They can be kept refrigerated for up to 2 months and are freezer friendly, for up to 6 months.

Nutrition

Serving: 1Heart | Calories: 95kcal | Carbohydrates: 7g | Protein: 5g | Fat: 6g | Fiber: 5g | Vitamin A: 4% | Vitamin C: 2% | Calcium: 3% | Iron: 2%

Easy Keto Fudge Recipe With Cocoa Powder & Sea Salt

Ingredients

- 1 cup Coconut oil (solid)
- 1/4 cup Powdered erythritol (to taste)
- 1/4 cup Cocoa powder
- 1 tsp Vanilla extract
- 1/8 tsp Sea salt
- Coarse sea salt flakes (optional - for topping)

Instructions

1. Line a 28 oz rectangular glass container with parchment paper, so that the parchment hangs out over the sides.

2. Using a hand mixer at LOW speed, beat the coconut oil and sweetener together, just until fluffy and combined.

3. Beat in the cocoa powder, vanilla and sea salt to taste. Adjust sweetener to taste. Do not overmix.

4. Transfer the mixture to the lined container. Smooth the top with a spatula or spoon.

5. Refrigerate the keto fudge for about 45-60 minutes, until solid.

6. Sprinkle the top of the fudge with sea salt flakes and press gently.

7. Run a knife along the edge and take out using the edges of the parchment paper. Slice carefully - see post above for slicing tips.

8. Keep the fudge refrigerated and bring to room temperature right before serving. You can also freeze it - see tips above. Do not leave at room temperature for prolonged periods, as it will melt easily.

Sopapilla Cheesecake Bars

Ingredients

Dough Ingredients:

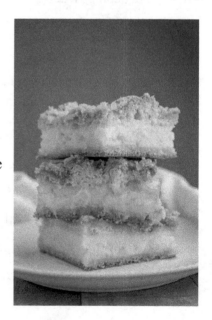

- 8 oz mozzarella shredded or cubed
- 2 oz cream cheese
- 1 egg
- 1/3 cup almond flour
- 1/3 cup coconut flour
- 2 tbsp Trim Healthy Mama Gentle Sweet or my sweetener
- 1 tsp vanilla
- 1 tsp baking powder

Cheesecake Filling Ingredients:

• 14 oz cream cheese

• 2 eggs

• 1/2 cup Trim Healthy Mama Gentle Sweet or my sweetener

• 1 tsp vanilla

Cinnamon Topping:

• 2 tbsp Trim Healthy Mama Gentle Sweet or my sweetener

• 1 tbsp cinnamon

• 2 tbsp melted butter

Instructions

1. Preheat oven to 350.

2. Put cheese in a microwave-safe bowl. Microwave one minute. Stir. Microwave 30 seconds. Stir. At this point, all the cheese should be melted. Microwave 30 more seconds until uniform and gloopy (it should look like cheese fondue at this point). Add the rest of the dough ingredients and the cheese to a food processor. Mix using the dough blade until a uniform color. Once it is a uniform color wet your hands and press half of it into an 8x8 baking dish. Press out the other half into an 8x8 square on a piece of parchment paper.

3. To make the cheesecake filling you can add the cream cheese, vanilla, eggs, and sweetener to the food processor (no need to wash) or to the bowl you were using. Mix until smooth in the food processor or with an electric mixer.

4. Pour the cheesecake batter on top of the bottom layer of dough. Gently put the other square of dough on top and peel off the parchment paper. Sprinkle the sweetener and cinnamon on top and drizzle with the melted butter.

5. Bake for 50-60 minutes until puffed up and golden brown. If the butter pools in the center you can brush it over the top with a pastry brush during the last 20 minutes of baking.

Recipe Notes

If you do not have a food processor you can mix in a medium bowl with a wooden spoon but you may need to dump it onto wax paper and knead it by hand to thoroughly incorporate the ingredients.

White Chocolate Peanut Butter Blondies

Ingredients

- 1/2 cup peanut butter
- 4 tbsp softened butter
- 2 eggs
- 1 tsp vanilla
- 3 tbsp melted raw cocoa butter
- 1/4 cup almond flour
- 1 tbsp coconut flour
- 1/2 cup Trim Healthy Mama Gentle Sweet or my sweetener
- 1/4 cup chopped raw cocoa butter

Instructions

1. Preheat oven to 350. Spray the bottom of a 9 x 9 baking dish with cooking spray.

2. With an electric mixer combine the first five ingredients until smooth. Add in the flours, sweetener, and chopped cocoa butter. Spread in the prepared baking dish. Bake for 25 minutes until the center no longer jiggles and the edges are golden.

3. Cool completely and then chill in the refrigerator for at least 2-3 hours before cutting.

Keto Espresso Chocolate Cheesecake Bars – Low Carb

Ingredients

For the chocolate crust:

• 7 tablespoons butter, melted

• 2 cups superfine, blanched almond flour (I used Honeyville)

• 3 tablespoons cocoa powder

• 1/3 cup granulated erythritol sweetener

For the cheesecake:

• 16 ounces full fat cream cheese

• 2 large eggs

• 1/2 cup granulated erythritol sweetener (I used Swerve)

• 2 tablespoons instant espresso powder (I used Cafe Bustelo)

• 1 teaspoon vanilla extract

• additional cocoa powder for dusting over the top if desired.

Instructions

For the chocolate crust:

1. Preheat the oven to 350° F.

2. Combine the melted butter, almond flour, sweetener and cocoa powder in a medium sized bowl and mix well.

3. Transfer the crust dough to a 9 x 9 pan lined with parchment paper or foil (this will make removing the bars much easier.)

4. Press the crust firmly into the bottom of the pan.

5. Bake the crust for 8 minutes.

6. Remove from the oven and set aside to cool.

For the cheesecake filling:

1. Combine the cream cheese, eggs, sweetener, espresso powder, and vanilla extract in a blender and blend until smooth.

2. Pour over the par baked crust and spread out evenly in the pan.

3. Bake the cheesecake bars at 350° F for 25 minutes, or until set.

4. Remove from the oven and cool.

5. Dust with optional cocoa powder if using.

6. Chill for at least 1 hour, preferably longer, before cutting into four rows of squares to serve.

7. Store in an airtight container in the refrigerator for up to 5 days, or freeze for up to 3 months.

Fudgy Keto Brownies

Ingredients

- 1/2 cup almond flour
- 1/4 cup cocoa powder
- 3/4 cup erythritol
- 1/2 tsp baking powder
- 1 tablespoon instant coffee optional
- 10 tablespoons butter 1/2 cup + 2 Tblsp
- 2 oz dark chocolate
- 3 eggs at room temperature
- ½ teaspoon vanilla extract optional

Instructions

1. Preheat oven to 350 degrees F (175 degrees C). Line an 8x8 inch or 8x9 pan with parchment paper, aluminum foil or grease with butter.

2. In a medium mixing bowl, whisk almond flour, cocoa powder, baking powder, erythritol, and instant coffee. Be sure to whisk out all the clumps from the erythritol.

3. In a large microwave-safe mixing bowl, Melt butter and chocolate for 30 seconds to 1 minute or until just melted. Whisk in the eggs and vanilla then gently whisk in the dry ingredients just until mixed through. Be careful not to over mix the batter or it will become cakey.

4. Transfer batter into a baking dish and bake for 18-20 minutes or until a toothpick inserted comes out moist. cool for at least 30 mins to 2 hours in the fridge and slice into 16 small squares.

Keto Donuts

Ingredients

- 2 large eggs room temperature
- 1/4 cup unsweetened almond milk
- 1/4 teaspoon apple cider vinegar
- 1 teaspoon vanilla extract
- 2 tablespoons melted ghee , OR butter if not paleo
- 1/4 cup granulated monkfruit sweetener , can also use SWERVE
- 1 cup super-fine blanched almond flour
- 1/2 tablespoon coconut flour
- 1/4 teaspoon xanthan gum
- 1 teaspoon ground cinnamon
- 1 1/2 teaspoons baking powder
- 1/2 teaspoon baking soda
- 1/8 fine sea salt
- mini donut pan

TOPPING CHOICES:

For the Cinnamon Sugar Coating:

- 1/4 cup granulated monkfruit , can also use granulated erythritol OR SWERVE

• 1 teaspoon ground cinnamon

• 1 1/2 tablespoons melted ghee , or buttter if not paleo

For the Chocolate Glaze:

• 2 ounces No sugar dark chocolate , melted

• 1 teaspoon coconut oil , melted

• 1 teaspoon powdered monkfruit sweetener

Instructions

1. In a large bowl, whisk together the eggs, almond milk, apple cider vinegar, melted ghee, vanilla, melted ghee & monk fruit sweetener, until smooth and combined.

2. In a separate medium bowl, combine the almond flour, coconut flour, xanthan gum, cinnamon, baking powder, baking soda and salt. Slowly add the dry ingredients to the wet ingredients & stir until just combined.

3. Transfer batter evenly into a greased 12 cavity silicone mini donut pan (or drop into mini muffin tins) (filling 3/4 full). (Or you can also use a 6 cavity silicone donut pan for regular-sized donuts.)

4. Bake in preheated oven 350F for 12-15 minutes (for mini) or (21-24 minutes for regular-sized) until golden brown.

Remove pan from the oven and set aside until the donuts are cool enough to handle.

FOR THE CINNAMON COATING:

1. While the donuts are baking, stir together the granulated sweetener and cinnamon in a small bowl.

In a separate small heat-safe bowl, melt ghee (or butter).

Take each cooled donut and lightly dunk in melted ghee then roll into the cinnamon/sweetener coating.

Repeat with remaining donuts.

FOR THE CHOCOLATE GLAZE:

1. Add the chopped chocolate and coconut oil to a small heat-safe bowl & melt in microwave. Stir in sweetener until combined.

Dip the cooled donuts into the chocolate (double-dip if you want a thicker glaze) and place in the fridge until the chocolate coating has set.

Healthy 1 Minute Low Carb Brownie

Ingredients

- 1 scoop chocolate protein powder 32-34 grams
- 1 tbsp coconut flour can substitute for gluten free oat flour
- 1 tbsp granulated sweetener Optional- I used a stevia blend
- 1/2 tsp baking powder
- 1 tbsp cocoa powder
- 1 egg white OR whole egg *
- 1/4 cup milk of choice **

• 1 tbsp chocolate chunks of choice Optional

Instructions

1. Lightly grease a small microwave safe cereal bowl or oven safe ramekin with cooking spray and set aside.

2. In a small mixing bowl, combine all your dry ingredients and mix well. Add your egg white, milk of choice and chocolate chunks and mix until a thick batter is formed. If the mixture is too thick (it will most likely be), continue to add milk, one tablespoon at a time, until a thick batter remains.

3. If using a microwave, microwave in 30-second intervals until desired texture is achieved (I usually get the best texture at 55 seconds). If using an oven, bake at 350 degrees Fahrenheit for 12-15 minutes, or until a skewer comes out 'just clean' from the center.

Notes

* To keep it vegan, omit completely- You'll need to add an extra tablespoon of non-dairy milk to compensate.

** Depending on the protein powder and coconut flour you use, you may need more. Adjust accordingly.

Mini Cinnamon Roll Cheesecakes

Ingredients

Crust

- 1/2 cup almond flour
- 2 tbsp Swerve Sweetener
- 1/2 tsp cinnamon
- 2 tbsp melted butter

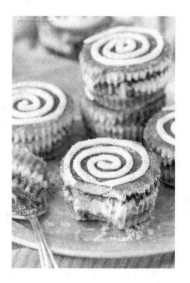

Cheesecake Filling

- 6 ounces cream cheese softened
- 5 tbsp Swerve Sweetener divided
- 1/4 cup sour cream
- 1/2 tsp vanilla extract
- 1 large egg
- 2 tsp cinnamon

Frosting

- 1 tbsp butter softened
- 3 tbsp confectioners Swerve Sweetener
- 1/4 tsp vanilla extract
- 2 tsp heavy cream

Instructions

Crust:

1. Preheat the oven to 325F and line a muffin pan with 6 parchment or silicone liners.

2. In a medium bowl, whisk together the almond flour, sweetener and cinnamon. Stir in the melted butter until the mixture begins to clump together.

3. Divide among the prepared muffin cups and press firmly into the bottom. Bake 7 minutes, then remove and let cool while preparing the filling.

Cheesecake Filling:

1. Reduce oven temperature to 300F. In a large bowl, beat the cream cheese and 3 tablespoons of the sweetener together until smooth. Beat in the sour cream, vanilla and egg until well combined.

2. In a small bowl, whisk together the remaining 2 tablespoons sweetener and the cinnamon.

3. Dollop about 3/4 tbsp of the cream cheese mixture into each of the muffin cups and sprinkle with a little of the cinnamon mixture. Repeat 2 more times. If you have any leftover cinnamon "sugar", reserve to sprinkle on after the cheesecakes are baked.

4. Bake 15 to 17 minutes, until mostly set but centres jiggle slightly. Turn off the oven and let them remain inside for 5 more minutes, then remove and let cool 30 minutes. Refrigerate at least 2 hours until set.

Frosting:

1. In a medium bowl, beat butter with powdered sweetener until well combined. Beat in vanilla extract and heavy cream.

2. Transfer to a small ziplock bag and snip the corner. Drizzle decoratively over the chilled cheesecakes.

Keto Chocolate Donuts

Ingredients

Donuts:

• Nonstick oil for pan

• 4 large eggs

• 1/2 cup unsalted butter, melted (112 grams)

• 3 tablespoons whole milk

• 1 teaspoon stevia glycerite (equals 1/3 cup sugar)

• ¼ cup coconut flour

• ¼ cup natural unsweetened cocoa powder (not treated with alkali)*

• ¼ teaspoon sea salt

• ¼ teaspoon baking soda

Glaze:

• 3/4 cup extra dark chocolate chips (4.5 oz)

• 1 tablespoon avocado oil

Instructions

1. Preheat oven to 350 degrees F. Grease 10 silicone donut pan cavities.

2. Whisk together the eggs, melted butter, milk and stevia.

3. Whisk in the coconut flour, cocoa powder, salt and baking soda.

4. Fill the donut pan cavities 3/4 full. Bake until set and a toothpick inserted in donuts comes out clean, about 17 minutes.

5. Place the pan on a cooling rack and allow to cool for 15 minutes.

6. Meanwhile, in a shallow bowl, melt the chocolate chips in the microwave, in 30-second intervals, stirring after each session. Stir in the avocado oil.

7. Gently run a knife around the edges and center of each donut. Carefully release the donuts from the pan. Dip each donut into the glaze. If desired, sprinkle with toppings such as shredded coconut or chopped nuts, or drizzle with melted peanut butter.

8. Cool the keto chocolate donuts until the glaze sets, about 30 minutes, then serve.

Notes

*The baking soda in this recipe needs an acid to react with, and cocoa powder treated with alkali will not provide that acid.
Nutrition label includes donuts and glaze, but no toppings.

Cheesy Biscuits / Scones

Ingredients

9 oz. 250g almond flour ground almonds (NOT almond meal)

½ tsp. salt

4 tsp. baking powder

1 tsp. xanthan gum

2 oz. / 55g butter

2 oz. / 55g sharp (strong) cheddar cheese, finely grated

⅓ cup / 2 ½ fl oz. unsweetened coconut or unsweetened almond milk

1 beaten egg to glaze

Instructions

1. Heat oven to 400°F.
2. Put the almond flour, other dry ingredients and butter in a food processor and pulse until it resembles fine breadcrumbs. You can also do this by hand if that's your thing.
3. Turn into a bowl and mix in the cheese until evenly distributed. Make a well in the center of the dry ingredients and pour in the milk.
4. Mix by hand to form a dough. It will be a little sticky.
5. Using almond flour to dust the surface, knead the dough lightly until smooth. Roll out the dough to ¾ inch thick.
6. Cut out biscuits using a round or fluted cutter.

7. Gather up the trimmings into a ball, re-roll and cut remaining dough into rounds. Place the scones on a baking sheet.

8. Brush tops with a beaten egg.

9. Bake for 8 – 10 minutes until golden brown.

Sour Cream and Chive Biscuits / Scones

Ingredients

15 oz. / 420g almond flour/ground almonds (NOT almond meal)

4 tsp. baking powder

1 tsp. baking soda

2 tsp. xanthan gum

½ tsp. salt

6 oz. / 170g unsalted butter, cold 1 egg

½ cup full-fat sour cream

1 TBSP cold water

½ oz. fresh chives, chopped

6 oz. / 170g full-fat feta cheese, chopped into small pieces Beaten egg to glaze Paprika

Instructions

1. Preheat oven to 375°F. Place almond flour, baking powder, baking soda, xanthan gum, salt, and cold butter into a food processor and pulse just until it resembles breadcrumbs. Do not over-process!

2. Turn into a mixing bowl and add the egg, sour cream, water, chives and feta cheese, and mix just enough to form a rough, soft dough. Turn onto a board and knead about 10 times until the dough comes together. It will be shaggy.

3. Flatten the dough lightly with your hand until it is a 1-inch thick square. Cut into 2-inch squares with a sharp knife.

4. Place biscuits on a baking sheet, brush with beaten egg and sprinkle with paprika.

5. Bake in the center of the oven for 12 – 15 minutes until golden brown.

Top Tip: Beware buying ready-crumbled feta cheese – it has corn or other starches in it to prevent the crumbles caking together. Instead, buy a piece of feta cheese and chop it into small pieces. Depending on your goals and where you are on your journey, if you want or need to reduce the fat, you can use low-fat versions of sour cream and feta.

Tomato Basil Biscuits / Scones

Ingredients

9 oz. 250g almond flour ground almonds (NOT almond meal)

½ tsp. salt

4 tsp. baking powder

1 tsp. xanthan gum

3 tsp. dried basil

2oz. / 55g butter **SUB: ghee for dairy-free**

2 oz. / 55g sun-dried tomatoes, pre-soaked in hot water to soften, drained, and then chopped

⅓ cup / 2 ½ fl oz. unsweetened coconut or unsweetened almond milk Beaten egg to glaze

Instructions

1. Heat oven to 400°F.
2. Put the almond flour, other dry ingredients, basil and butter in a food processor and pulse until it resembles fine breadcrumbs. You can also do this by hand if that's your thing.

3. Turn into a bowl and mix in the sun-dried tomatoes until evenly distributed. Make a well in the center of the dry ingredients and pour in the milk.

4. Mix by hand to form a dough. Knead the dough lightly until smooth. Divide dough into eight 2 oz. / 55g pieces of dough.

5. Roll each piece in your hands to make a ball, please on baking sheet and flatten gently to resemble a cookie.

6. Brush tops with beaten egg.

7. Bake for 10 minutes until golden brown.

8. Carefully use a serrated knife to cut open, especially if they are still warm, as they are quite fragile.

If you like tomatoes, these biscuits will send you into a complete dither. In a good way.

Collagen Keto Bread

Ingredients:

1/2 cup Unflavored Grass-Fed Collagen Protein

6 tablespoons almond flour (see recipe notes below for nut-free substitute)

5 pastured eggs, separated

1 tablespoon unflavored liquid coconut oil

1 teaspoon aluminum-free baking powder

1 teaspoon xanthan gum (see recipe notes for substitute)

Pinch Himalayan pink salt

Optional: a pinch of stevia

Instructions:

Preheat oven to 325 degrees F.

Generously oil only the bottom part of a standard size (1.5 quarts) glass or ceramic loaf dish with coconut oil (or butter or ghee). Or you may use a piece of parchment paper trimmed to fit the bottom of your dish. Not oiling or lining the sides of your dish will allow the bread to attach to the sides and stay lifted while it cools.

In a large bowl, beat the egg whites until stiff peaks form. Set aside.

In a small bowl, whisk the dry ingredients together and set aside. Add the optional pinch of stevia if you're not a fan of eggs. It'll help offset the flavor without adding sweetness to your loaf.

In a small bowl, whisk together the wet ingredients — egg yolks and liquid coconut oil — and set aside.

Add the dry and the wet ingredients to the egg whites and mix until well incorporated. Your batter will be thick and a little gooey.

Pour the batter into the oiled or lined dish and place in the oven.

Bake for 40 minutes. The bread will rise significantly in the oven.

Remove from oven and let it cool completely — about 1 to 2 hours. The bread will sink some and that's OK.

Once the bread is cooled, run the sharp edge of a knife around the edges of the dish to release the loaf.

Slice into 12 even slices.

Important Notes:

Storing Leftovers: Store loosely covered in the refrigerator for up to 5 days.

Reheating: You can eat this bread cold (it stays nice and moist), or bring to room temperature by setting it out on the counter, or pan-sear on the stovetop with ghee or butter. I don't recommend toasting it in a toaster. Although it does work, it's not my preferred method as it tends to dry out too quickly.

Tasting Notes: To set expectations correctly, you should understand that this is not gluten bread nor is it Paleo bread, both of which generally have a fair amount of carbs, often coming from starches and sugars. Rather, this is an extremely low carb/zero carb keto bread alternative. With that said, you may taste eggs, especially if you're not a fan of their flavor. Additionally, the texture is lighter than gluten bread and won't have the "chew" you may be accustomed to. However, if you're a seasoned keto bread eater, I think you'll find this to be a wonderful option.

Recipe Notes: For those that can't tolerate almond flour, substitute the same amount of coconut flour and add 3 tablespoons of full-fat canned coconut milk (BPA-free) to your ingredients list (you will add coconut milk when instructions call for mixing wet ingredients). This will increase the net carbs by 1.5 grams per serving and will make a more dense texture. For keto bread without xanthan gum, substitute with 3/4 tablespoon of konjac flour (also known as glucomannan powder). This will not change the net carb count.

Nutritional Information: Calories: 77 | Protein: 7g | Carbs: 1g | Fiber: 1g | Sugar: 0g | Sugar Alcohol:0g | Net Carbs: 0g | Fat: 5g | Saturated Fat: 2g | Polyunsaturated: 0g | Monounsaturated: 1g | Trans fat: 0g | Cholesterol: 77g | Sodium: 86mg | Potassium: 51mg | Vitamin A: 3% | Vitamin C: 0% | Calcium: 4% | Iron: 3%

Best Keto Bread

Ingredients

1 1/2 Cup Almond Flour

6 Large eggs Separated

1/4 cup butter melted

3 tsp Baking powder

1/4 tsp Cream of Tartar It's ok if you don't have this

1 pinch pink Himalayan salt

6 drops Liquid Stevia optional

Instructions

1. Preheat oven to 375.

Separate the egg whites from the yolks. Add Cream of Tartar to the whites and beat until soft peaks are achieved.

In a food processor combine the egg yolks, 1/3 of the beaten egg whites, melted butter, almond flour, baking powder and salt (Adding ~6 drops of liquid stevia to the batter can help reduce the mild egg taste). Mix until combined. This will be a lumpy thick dough until the whites are added.

Add the remaining 2/3 of the egg whites and gently process until fully incorporated. Be careful not to overmix as this is what gives the bread it's volume!

Pour mixture into a buttered 8x4 loaf pan. Bake for 30 minutes. Check with a toothpick to ensure the bread is cooked through. Enjoy! 1 loaf makes 20 slices.

Nutrition

Serving: 25g | Calories: 90kcal | Carbohydrates: 2g | Protein: 3g | Fat: 7g | Fiber: 0.75g

Paleo Coconut Bread

Ingredients

1/2 cup coconut flour

1/4 tsp salt

1/4 tsp baking soda

6 eggs

¼ cup coconut oil, melted

¼ unsweetened almond milk

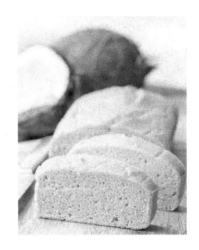

Directions

Preheat oven to 350°F.

Line an 8×4 inch loaf pan with parchment paper.

In a bowl combine the coconut flour, baking soda, and salt.

In another bowl combine the eggs, milk, and oil.

Slowly add the wet ingredients into the dry ingredients and mix until combined.

Pour the mixture into the prepared loaf pan.

Bake for 40-50 minutes, or until a toothpick, inserted in the middle comes out clean.

Easy Paleo Keto Bread Recipe

Ingredients

Basic Ingredients

1 cup Blanched almond flour

1/4 cup Coconut flour

2 tsp Gluten-free baking powder

1/4 tsp Sea salt

1/3 cup butter (or 5 tbsp + 1 tsp; measured solid, then melted; can use coconut oil for dairy-free)

12 large Egg white (~1 1/2 cups, at room temperature)

Optional Ingredients (recommended)

1 1/2 tbsp Erythritol (can use any sweetener or omit)

1/4 tsp Xanthan gum (for texture - omit for paleo)

1/4 tsp Cream of tartar (to more easily whip egg whites)

Instructions

1. Preheat the oven to 325 degrees F (163 degrees C). Line an 8 1/2 x 4 1/2 in (22x11 cm) loaf pan with parchment paper, with extra hanging over the sides for easy removal later.

2. Combine the almond flour, coconut flour, baking powder, erythritol, xanthan gum, and sea salt in a large food processor. Pulse until combined.

3. Add the melted butter. Pulse, scraping down the sides as needed, until crumbly.

4. In a very large bowl, use a hand mixer to beat the egg whites and cream of tartar (if using), until stiff peaks form. Make sure the bowl is large enough because the whites will expand a lot.

5. Add 1/2 of the stiff egg whites to the food processor. Pulse a few times until just combined. Do not over-mix!

6. Carefully transfer the mixture from the food processor into the bowl with the egg whites, and gently fold until no streaks remain. Do not stir. Fold gently to keep the mixture as fluffy as possible.

7. Transfer the batter to the lined loaf pan and smooth the top. Push the batter toward the center a bit to round the top.

8. Bake for about 40 minutes, until the top is golden brown. Tent the top with aluminum foil and bake for another 30-45 minutes, until the top is firm and does not make a squishy sound when pressed. Internal temperature should be 200 degrees. Cool completely before removing from the pan and slicing.

Dairy-free Paleo Cloud Bread Recipe

Ingredients

3 eggs

3 tbsp coconut cream spoon from a refrigerated can of full-fat coconut milk

1/2 tsp baking powder

optional toppings: sea salt black pepper and rosemary or whatever seasonings you like!

Instructions

1. Firstly, prep everything. Once you start going, you'll need to move quickly so have everything handy. Pre-heat the oven to 325f degrees and arrange a rack in the middle. Line a baking sheet with parchment paper and set aside. Grab your tools: hand mixer (you can use a stand mixer, but I find it to be better for

whipping egg whites so I can stay in control), all ingredients, any additional seasonings, two mixing bowls (the larger one should be used for egg whites), a large spoon to scoop and drop the bread with.

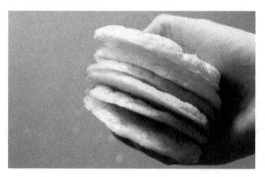

2. Using a full-fat can of coconut milk that has been refrigerated overnight or several hours, spoon out the top coconut cream and add to the smaller bowl.

3. Separate eggs into the two bowls, adding the yolk to the bowl with the cream and be careful to not let the yolk get into the whites in the larger bowl.

4. Using a hand mixer, beat the yolk and cream together first until nice and creamy, make sure there are no clumps of coconut left.

5. Wash your whisks well and dry them.

6. Add the baking powder into the whites and start beating on medium with the hand mixer for a few minutes, moving around and you'll see it get firmer. Keep going for a few minutes, you want to get it as thick as you can with stiff peaks. The thicker the better. Just don't over-do it. Once you can stop and dip the whisks in leaving peaks behind, you're ready.

7. Quickly and carefully add the yolk-coconut mixture into the whites, folding with a spatula, careful not to deflate too much. Keep going until everything is well combined but still fluffy.

8. Now you can grab your spoon and start dropping your batter down on the baking sheet. Keep going as quickly and carefully as you can, or it will start to melt. They should look pillowy.

9. Steadily add your baking sheet to the middle rack in the oven and bake for approx. 20-25 minutes. You should be able to scoop them up with your spatula and see a fluffy top and a flat bottom. Store in the fridge for about a week or freeze.

Keto Pecan Cookies

Ingredients

2 cups almond flour

2 tablespoons Erythritol

1/2 teaspoon Baking Powder

4 ounces Unsalted Butter softened

1 Egg

1 teaspoon vanilla essence

2 tablespoons Sugar-Free Maple Syrup

16 pecan halves

US Customary - Metric

Instructions

1. Preheat your oven to 160C/320F and prepare your cookie sheet by lining with parchment paper.

2. In your food processor add the almond flour, natvia, baking powder, and butter. Pulse until the mixture starts to stick together.

3. Add the egg, vanilla, and Sugar-Free Maple Syrup and blend until it is all combined.

4. Scrape the mixture out into a mixing bowl, and roll together using your hands (we find food-safe gloves great for keeping your hands clean). If the dough is too sticky, add an extra tablespoon of almond flour and gently knead through.

5. Split the dough in half and each half into 8 evenly sized pieces, roll each piece into a ball and gently press onto your prepared cookie sheet. The cookies do not spread and will retain almost the same shape that you press them into.

6. Press a pecan half into the center of each cookie.

7. Bake in the oven for 15-20 minutes. They are cooked when golden brown with firm edges.

8. Allow cooling before enjoying.

Nutrition

Serving: 1cookie | Calories: 147kcal | Carbohydrates: 4g | Protein: 3g | Fat: 13g | Saturated Fat: 4g | Cholesterol: 25mg | Sodium: 8mg | Potassium: 22mg | Fiber: 2g | Sugar: 1g | Vitamin A: 190IU | Calcium: 39mg | Iron: 0.6mg

Keto Snickerdoodle Cookies

Ingredients

3/4 cup almond meal

1 tablespoon cream of tartar

2 teaspoons Baking Powder

2 tablespoons cinnamon ground

1/2 cup natvia

14 ounces Walnut Butter

3 eggs

1 tablespoon natvia icing mix for rolling

2 teaspoons cinnamon for rolling

Instructions

1. Preheat fan-forced oven to 180C/350F.
2. In a bowl add the almond meal, cream of tartar, baking powder, cinnamon, and natvia and stir until combined.
3. Add the walnut butter and eggs to the dry ingredients and mix well. The dough will be very thick and sticky.
4. In a separate bowl mix the natvia icing mix and 2 teaspoons of cinnamon.
5. Take tablespoon-sized scoops of the cookie dough and roll into balls. We used disposable gloves to handle the sticky dough and it makes clean up a breeze.

6. Flatten the balls to your desired cookie thickness, we made ours 1/4in/7mm thick. Press the flattened dough into the cinnamon and icing mixture and coat all sides.

7. Place the coated cookies onto a lined cookie pan. The cookies do not spread and can be placed close together.

8. Bake for 10-12 minutes. Cookies are done when the edges feel firm and are starting to brown. They will harden up as they cool.

We love our cookies still warm, but they'll keep for at least 1 week in an airtight container. Enjoy.

Nutrition

Serving: 1cookie | Calories: 128kcal | Carbohydrates: 4g | Protein: 3g | Fat: 12g | Saturated Fat: 1g | Polyunsaturated Fat: 6g | Monounsaturated Fat: 1g | Sodium: 1mg | Potassium: 147mg | Fiber: 2g | Sugar: 1g | Vitamin C: 0.8mg | Calcium: 40mg | Iron: 1.1mg

Keto Macadamia Nut Cookies

Ingredients

350 g macadamia butter homemade

75 g almond meal

2 eggs

70 g Xylitol

1 tsp vanilla extract

1 tsp cinnamon

Instructions

1. Preheat fan-forced oven to 320F/160C.
2. Mix all ingredients in a bowl.
3. Roll into teaspoon-sized balls and press onto a lined baking tray. The cookies will need to be pressed into their desired shape as they have minimal spreading. They can be placed quite close together.
4. Bake the cookies in the preheated oven for 12 minutes or until golden brown, with the edges starting to harden. The cookies with continue to harden as they cool.

Nutrition

Calories: 132kcal | Carbohydrates: 3g | Protein: 2g | Fat: 13g | Saturated Fat: 2g | Polyunsaturated Fat: 0.2g | Monounsaturated Fat: 9g | Sodium: 1mg | Potassium: 54mg | Fiber: 2g | Sugar: 1g | Vitamin C: 0.2mg | Calcium: 20mg | Iron: 0.7mg

Keto Wafers

Ingredients

2.83 large egg whites

3.31 ounces unsweetened shredded coconut

0.24 cup Erythritol

0.94 pinch Salt

2.83 tbsp butter melted

11.33 drops Liquid Stevia

Instructions

Preheat fan-forced oven to 150C/300F.

In a bowl mix the egg whites, coconut, Natvia and salt. Mix well.

Add the melted butter and mix well.

FOR ROUND WAFERS: Drop tablespoon-sized balls onto a lined cookie sheet and press down until they are 1/4in/5mm thick

FOR WAFER SHARDS: Pour the mix onto a lined cookie sheet, place parchment paper over the top and roll into a 1/4in/5mm thick sheet. Using a knife, gently press lines into the sheet to split the wafers later on.

Bake both types of wafers in the oven for 20 mins, then turn the tray around and bake for another 5 minutes. Remove when the edges are browned.

The wafers will appear soft immediately after baking, allow to sit for 10 minutes to harden up. If your wafers are too thick they may require additional cooking time.

Once cooled, wafers can be stored in an airtight container to retain their crunch.

Nutrition

Serving: 1wafer | Calories: 57kcal | Carbohydrates: 2g | Protein: 1g | Fat: 6g | Saturated Fat: 5g | Polyunsaturated Fat: 0.1g | Monounsaturated Fat: 1g | Cholesterol: 5mg | Sodium: 11mg | Potassium: 10mg | Fiber: 1g | Sugar: 0.4g | Vitamin A: 50IU | Calcium: 0.5mg | Iron: 0.2mg

Garlic & Herb Focaccia

Ingredients

Dry Ingredients

1 cup Almond Flour

¼ cup Coconut Flour

½ tsp Xanthan Gum

1 tsp Garlic Powder

1 tsp Flaky Salt

½ tsp Baking Soda

½ tsp Baking Powder

Wet Ingredients

2 eggs

1 tbsp Lemon Juice

2 tsp Olive oil + 2 tbsp Olive Oil to drizzle

Top with Italian Seasoning and TONS of flaky salt!

Instructions

1. Heat oven to 350 and line a baking tray or 8-inch round pan with parchment.

2. Whisk together the dry ingredients making sure there are no lumps.

3. Beat the egg, lemon juice, and oil until combined.

4. Mix the wet and the dry together, working quickly, and scoop the dough into your pan.

***Make sure not to mix the wet and dry until you are ready to put the bread in the oven because the leavening reaction begins once it is mixed!!!

Smooth the top and edges with a spatula dipped in water (or your hands) then use your finger to dimple the dough. Don't be afraid to go deep on the dimples! Again, a little water keeps it from sticking.

Bake covered for about 10 minutes. Drizzle with Olive Oil bake for an additional 10-15 minutes uncovering to brown gently.

Top with more flaky salt, olive oil (optional), a dash of Italian seasoning and fresh basil. Let cool completely before slicing for optimal texture!!

Notes

3g Net Carbs per big long slice.

You can also cut it into squares and you'd just want to adjust how many servings you get vs the macros1

Nutrition Information

Serving size: 1 Calorie: 166 Fat: 13 Carbohydrates: 7 Fiber: 4 Protein: 7

Cauliflower Bread with Garlic & Herbs

Ingredients

3 cup Cauliflower ("riced" using food processor*)

10 large Egg (separated)

1/4 tsp Cream of tartar (optional)

1 1/4 cup Coconut flour

1 1/2 tbsp Gluten-free baking powder

1 tsp Sea salt

6 tbsp Butter (unsalted, measured solid, then melted; can use ghee for dairy-free)

6 cloves Garlic (minced)

1 tbsp fresh rosemary (chopped)

1 tbsp Fresh parsley (chopped)

Instructions

1. Preheat the oven to 350 degrees F (177 degrees C). Line a 9x5 in (23x13 cm) loaf pan with parchment paper.

2. Steam the riced cauliflower. You can do this in the microwave (cooked for 3-4 minutes, covered in plastic) OR in a steamer basket over water on the stove (line with cheesecloth if the holes in the steamer basket are too big, and steam for a few minutes). Both ways, steam until the cauliflower is soft and tender. Allow the cauliflower to cool enough to handle.

3. Meanwhile, use a hand mixer to beat the egg whites and cream of tartar until stiff peaks form.

4. Place the coconut flour, baking powder, sea salt, egg yolks, melted butter, garlic, and 1/4 of the whipped egg whites in a food processor.

5. When the cauliflower has cooled enough to handle, wrap it in a kitchen towel and squeeze several times to release as much moisture as possible. (This is important - the end result should be very dry and clump together.) Add the cauliflower to the food processor. Process until well combined. (Mixture will be dense and a little crumbly.)

6. Add the remaining egg whites to the food processor. Fold in just a little, to make it easier to process. Pulse a few times until just incorporated. (Mixture will be fluffy.) Fold in the chopped parsley and rosemary. (Don't overmix to avoid breaking down the egg whites too much.)

7. Transfer the batter into the lined baking pan. Smooth the top and round slightly. If desired, you can press more herbs into the top (optional).

8. Bake for about 45-50 minutes, until the top is golden. Cool completely before removing and slicing.

How To Make Buttered Low Carb Garlic Bread (optional): Top slices generously with butter, minced garlic, fresh parsley, and a little sea salt. Bake in a preheated oven at 450 degrees F (233 degrees C) for about 10 minutes. If you want it more browned, place under the broiler for a couple of minutes.

You'll need to use the food processor twice - first to rice the cauliflower and then again to mix everything together. No need to wash in between, just rinse lightly to get rid of the raw cauliflower florets stuck to the sides.

15-Minute Gluten Free & Keto Tortillas

Ingredients

96 g almond flour

24 g coconut flour

2 teaspoons xanthan gum

1 teaspoon baking powder

1/4 teaspoon kosher salt

2 teaspoons apple cider vinegar

1 egg lightly beaten

3 teaspoons water

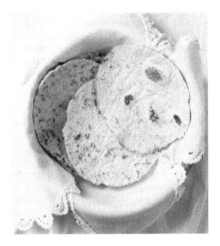

Instructions

1.   Add almond flour, coconut flour, xanthan gum, baking powder and salt to a food processor. Pulse until thoroughly combined. Note: you can alternatively whisk everything in a large bowl and use a hand or stand mixer for the following steps.

2.   Pour in apple cider vinegar with the food processor running. Once it has distributed evenly, pour in the egg. Followed by the water. Stop the food processor once the dough forms into a ball. The dough will be sticky to touch.

3.   Wrap dough in cling film and knead it through the plastic for a minute or two. Think of it a bit like a stress ball. Allow dough to rest for 10 minutes (and up to three days in the fridge).

4.   Heat up a skillet (preferably) or pan over medium heat. You can test the heat by sprinkling a few water droplets if the drops evaporate immediately your pan is too hot. The droplets should 'run' through the skillet.

5.   Break the dough into eight 1" balls (26g each). Roll out between two sheets of parchment or waxed paper with a rolling pin or using a tortilla press (easier!) until each round is 5-inches in diameter.

6.   Transfer to skillet and cook over medium heat for just 3-6 seconds (very important). Flip it over immediately (using a thin spatula or knife), and continue to cook until just lightly golden on each side (though with the traditional charred marks), 30 to 40 seconds. The key is not to overcook them, as they will no longer be pliable or puff up.

7.   Keep them warm wrapped in kitchen cloth until serving. To rewarm, heat briefly on both sides until just warm (less than a minute).

8.   These tortillas are best eaten straight away. But feel free to keep some dough handy in your fridge for up to three days, and they also freeze well for up to three months.

Cauliflower Tortillas

Ingredients

3/4 large head cauliflower (or two cups riced)

2 large eggs (Vegans, sub flax eggs)

1/4 cup chopped fresh cilantro

1/2 medium lime, juiced and zested

salt & pepper, to taste

Instructions

1. Preheat the oven to 375 degrees F., and line a baking sheet with parchment paper.

2. Trim the cauliflower, cut it into small, uniform pieces, and pulse in a food processor in batches until you get a couscous-like consistency. The finely riced cauliflower should make about 2 cups packed.

3. Place the cauliflower in a microwave-safe bowl and microwave for 2 minutes, then stir and microwave again for another 2 minutes. If you don't use a microwave, a steamer works just as well. Place the cauliflower in a fine cheesecloth or thin dishtowel and squeeze out as much liquid as possible, being careful not to burn yourself. Dishwashing gloves are suggested as it is very hot.

4. In a medium bowl, whisk the eggs. Add in cauliflower, cilantro, lime, salt, and pepper. Mix until well combined. Use your hands to shape 6 small "tortillas" on the parchment paper.

5. Bake for 10 minutes, carefully flip each tortilla and return to the oven for an additional 5 to 7 minutes, or until completely set. Place tortillas on a wire rack to cool slightly.

6. Heat a medium-sized skillet on medium. Place a baked tortilla in the pan, pressing down slightly, and brown for 1 to 2 minutes on each side. Repeat with remaining tortillas.

Buttery & Soft Skillet Flatbread

Ingredients

1 cup Almond Flour

2 tbsp Coconut Flour

2 tsp Xanthan Gum

1/2 tsp Baking Powder

1/2 tsp Falk Salt

1 Whole Egg + 1 Egg White

1 tbsp Water

1 tbsp Oil for frying

1 tbsp melted Butter-for slathering

Instructions

1. Whisk together the dry ingredients (flours, xanthan gum, baking powder, salt) until well combined.

2. Add the egg and egg white and beat gently into the flour to incorporate. The dough will begin to form.

3. Add the tablespoon of water and begin to work the dough to allow the flour and xanthan gum to absorb the moisture.
4. Cut the dough in 4 equal parts and press each section out with cling wrap. Watch the video for instructions!
5. Heat a large skillet over medium heat and add oil.
6. Fry each flatbread for about 1 min on each side.
7. Brush with butter (while hot) and garnish with salt and chopped parsley.

Fluffy Keto Almond Flour Biscuits

Ingredients:

1 cup almond flour

1/8 cup grass-fed ghee, melted

1 egg

1/2 teaspoon salt

1/4 teaspoon pepper

1/4 teaspoon garlic powder

1/2 teaspoon baking soda

1/2 tablespoon apple cider vinegar

1/2 cup basil (loosely packed), 1/2 teaspoon matcha, or your favorite herbs and spices (optional)

Instructions:

1. Preheat your oven to 350 degrees. Line a baking sheet with parchment.

2. If you make almond flour biscuits plain, mix all ingredients together in a mixing bowl and proceed to step 3. If using basil or matcha, blend almond flour, matcha, and basil together in a blender until well combined. Then, mix in remaining ingredients until a batter forms. If the mixture doesn't seem doughy enough when you roll it gently in your hands, add in an extra almond meal (1 tablespoon at a time, up to 3 tablespoons) until it forms a dough.

3. Scoop the dough out and form 7 balls. Place onto your prepared baking sheet and flatten each one slightly with the palm of your hand.

4. Bake for 15 minutes, or slightly golden and firm, but soft on the inside.

5. Remove biscuits from the oven and cool completely on a wire rack.

6. Enjoy warm, or store in a covered container and reheat gently later.

Nutritional Information: Calories: 151 | Fat: 14.6g | Salt: 187mg | Carbs: 3.1g | Fiber: 1.7g | Sugar: .6g | Protein: 3.7g | Cholesterol: 23mg | Net Carbs: 1.4g | Potassium: 121mg | Vitamin D: 2mcg | Calcium: 40mg | Iron: 1mg

Fluffy Keto Buns

Ingredients:

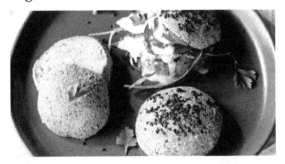

1/4 cup coconut flour

2 tablespoons ground psyllium husks

4 egg whites

2 egg yolks

1 teaspoon paleo baking powder

1/2 tablespoon apple cider vinegar

1 cup of water

1 teaspoon dried oregano (optional)

1 teaspoon dried thyme (optional)

Salt and pepper to taste

Instructions:

1. Preheat your oven to 350 degrees. Line a baking sheet with parchment paper.
2. With a hand mixer or whisk, beat the egg whites until they form a foam with stiff peaks. Set aside.
3. Mix all remaining ingredients in a separate bowl. Gently fold in the egg whites.

4. Form four thick, evenly sized rolls from your dough and place on the baking sheet. (Thickness is important so buns don't flatten.)

5. Bake for 40 minutes, or until cooked all the way through. If you cut one open and it still is moist, place them (even the one you have cut open) back in the oven for a few more minutes.

6. Remove from your oven and serve warm.

Nutritional Information : Calories: 120 | Fat: 3.1g | Salt: 121mg | Carbs: 23.4g | Fiber: 17.3gg | Sugar: 0.3g | Net Carbs: 6.1g | Protein: 6g | Cholesterol: 105mg | Potassium: 203mg | Calcium: 80mg | Iron: 1mg

Keto Pecan Cookies

Ingredients

2 cups almond flour

2 tablespoons Erythritol

1/2 teaspoon Baking Powder

4 ounces Unsalted Butter softened

1 Egg

1 teaspoon vanilla essence

2 tablespoons Sugar-Free Maple Syrup

16 pecan halves

US Customary - Metric

Instructions

1. Preheat your oven to 160C/320F and prepare your cookie sheet by lining with parchment paper.
2. In your food processor add the almond flour, natvia, baking powder, and butter. Pulse until the mixture starts to stick together.
3. Add the egg, vanilla, and Sugar-Free Maple Syrup and blend until it is all combined.
4. Scrape the mixture out into a mixing bowl, and roll together using your hands (we find food-safe gloves great for keeping your hands clean). If the dough is too sticky, add an extra tablespoon of almond flour and gently knead through.
5. Split the dough in half and each half into 8 evenly sized pieces, roll each piece into a ball and gently press onto your prepared cookie sheet. The cookies do not spread and will retain almost the same shape that you press them into.
6. Press a pecan half into the center of each cookie.
7. Bake in the oven for 15-20 minutes. They are cooked when golden brown with firm edges.
8. Allow cooling before enjoying.

Nutrition

Serving: 1cookie | Calories: 147kcal | Carbohydrates: 4g | Protein: 3g | Fat: 13g | Saturated Fat: 4g | Cholesterol: 25mg | Sodium: 8mg | Potassium: 22mg | Fiber: 2g | Sugar: 1g | Vitamin A: 190IU | Calcium: 39mg | Iron: 0.6mg

Keto Snickerdoodle Cookies

Ingredients

3/4 cup almond meal

1 tablespoon cream of tartar

2 teaspoons Baking Powder

2 tablespoons cinnamon ground

1/2 cup natvia

14 ounces Walnut Butter

3 eggs

1 tablespoon natvia icing mix for rolling

2 teaspoons cinnamon for rolling

Instructions

1. Preheat fan-forced oven to 180C/350F.
2. In a bowl add the almond meal, cream of tartar, baking powder, cinnamon, and natvia and stir until combined.
3. Add the walnut butter and eggs to the dry ingredients and mix well. The dough will be very thick and sticky.
4. In a separate bowl mix the natvia icing mix and 2 teaspoons of cinnamon.
5. Take tablespoon-sized scoops of the cookie dough and roll into balls. We used disposable gloves to handle the sticky dough and it makes clean up a breeze.
6. Flatten the balls to your desired cookie thickness, we made ours 1/4in/7mm thick. Press the flattened dough into the cinnamon and icing mixture and coat all sides.

7. Place the coated cookies onto a lined cookie pan. The cookies do not spread and can be placed close together.

Bake for 10-12 minutes. Cookies are done when the edges feel firm and are starting to brown. They will harden up as they cool.

We love our cookies still warm, but they'll keep for at least 1 week in an airtight container. Enjoy.

Nutrition

Serving: 1cookie | Calories: 128kcal | Carbohydrates: 4g | Protein: 3g | Fat: 12g | Saturated Fat: 1g | Polyunsaturated Fat: 6g | Monounsaturated Fat: 1g | Sodium: 1mg | Potassium: 147mg | Fiber: 2g | Sugar: 1g | Vitamin C: 0.8mg | Calcium: 40mg | Iron: 1.1mg

Keto Macadamia Nut Cookies

Ingredients

350 g macadamia butter homemade

75 g almond meal

2 eggs

70 g Xylitol

1 tsp vanilla extract

1 tsp cinnamon

Instructions

1. Preheat fan-forced oven to 320F/160C.

2. Mix all ingredients in a bowl.

3. Roll into teaspoon-sized balls and press onto a lined baking tray. The cookies will need to be pressed into their desired shape as they have minimal spreading. They can be placed quite close together.

4. Bake the cookies in the preheated oven for 12 minutes or until golden brown, with the edges starting to harden. The cookies with continue to harden as they cool.

Nutrition

Calories: 132kcal | Carbohydrates: 3g | Protein: 2g | Fat: 13g | Saturated Fat: 2g | Polyunsaturated Fat: 0.2g | Monounsaturated Fat: 9g | Sodium: 1mg | Potassium: 54mg | Fiber: 2g | Sugar: 1g | Vitamin C: 0.2mg | Calcium: 20mg | Iron: 0.7mg

Keto Wafers

Ingredients

2.83 large egg whites

3.31 ounces unsweetened shredded coconut

0.24 cup Erythritol

0.94 pinch Salt

2.83 tbsp butter melted

11.33 drops Liquid Stevia

Instructions

Preheat fan-forced oven to 150C/300F.

In a bowl mix the egg whites, coconut, Natvia and salt. Mix well.

Add the melted butter and mix well.

FOR ROUND WAFERS: Drop tablespoon-sized balls onto a lined cookie sheet and press down until they are 1/4in/5mm thick

FOR WAFER SHARDS: Pour the mix onto a lined cookie sheet, place parchment paper over the top and roll into a 1/4in/5mm thick sheet. Using a knife, gently press lines into the sheet to split the wafers later on.

Bake both types of wafers in the oven for 20 mins, then turn the tray around and bake for another 5 minutes. Remove when the edges are browned.

The wafers will appear soft immediately after baking, allow to sit for 10 minutes to harden up. If your wafers are too thick they may require additional cooking time.

Once cooled, wafers can be stored in an airtight container to retain their crunch.

Nutrition

Serving: 1wafer | Calories: 57kcal | Carbohydrates: 2g | Protein: 1g | Fat: 6g | Saturated Fat: 5g | Polyunsaturated Fat: 0.1g | Monounsaturated Fat: 1g | Cholesterol: 5mg | Sodium: 11mg | Potassium: 10mg | Fiber: 1g | Sugar: 0.4g | Vitamin A: 50IU | Calcium: 0.5mg | Iron: 0.2mg

Drop Biscuits

Ingredients

1 egg

77 g sour cream or coconut cream + 2 tsp. apple cider vinegar, at room temp

2 tablespoons water

1 tablespoon apple cider vinegar

96 g almond flour

63 g golden flaxseed meal or psyllium husk, finely ground

21 g coconut flour

20 g whey protein isolate or more almond flour

3 1/2 teaspoons baking powder

1 teaspoon xanthan gum or 1 TBS. flaxseed meal

1/2 teaspoon kosher salt

112 g organic grass-fed butter or 7 TBS. ghee/coconut oil

Instructions

1. Preheat oven to 450°F/230°C. Line a baking tray with parchment paper or a baking mat.

2. Add eggs, sour (or coconut) cream, water, and apple cider vinegar to a medium bowl and whisk for a minute or two until fully mixed. Set aside.

3. Add almond flour, flaxseed meal, coconut flour, whey protein, baking powder, xanthan gum (or more flax) and kosher salt to a food processor and pulse until very thoroughly combined.

4. Add in the butter and pulse a few times until pea-sized. Pour in the egg and cream mixture, pulsing until combined. The dough will be very shaggy.

5. Drop 6 rounds of dough onto the prepared baking tray. Brush with melted butter and bake for 15-20 minutes until deep golden. Allow cooling for 10 minutes before serving. These guys keep well, stored in an airtight container at room temperature, for 3-4 days.

6. You can freeze the shaped biscuit dough for 1-2 months, and bake straight from the freezer as needed.

Turmeric Cauliflower Buns

Ingredients

1 medium head of cauliflower or about 2 cups of firmly packed cauliflower rice (see directions for making the cauliflower rice)

2 eggs

2 tablespoons coconut flour

¼ teaspoon ground turmeric

pinch each of salt and pepper

Instructions

1. Preheat oven to 400°F.

2. Line a baking sheet with parchment paper and set aside.

3. Take your cauliflower and use a sharp knife to cut off the base. Pull off any green parts and use your hands to break the

cauliflower into florets. Give the florets a quick rinse and pat dry.

4. Next, make cauliflower rice by placing the florets into the bowl of a food processor with the "S" blade. Pulse for about 30 seconds until the cauliflower is about the size of rice. You should have about two cups of firmly packed cauliflower rice.

5. Place the cauliflower rice into a microwavable-safe bowl with about a teaspoon of water. Cover with plastic wrap and poke a few holes to let the steam escape. Microwave the cauliflower rice for about 3 minutes. Alternatively, you can steam the cauliflower rice on the stovetop in a steamer basket.

6. Uncover the bowl and let the cauliflower rice cool for about 5 minutes. Then, use a large spoon to put the cauliflower rice into a nut milk bag or a clean dish towel. Squeeze the excess moisture out, being careful not to burn your hands.

7. Pour the cauliflower rice into a medium mixing bowl and stir in the eggs, turmeric, and a pinch of salt and black pepper.

8. Use your hands to form the mixture into 6 buns, placing them on the baking sheet.

9. Bake for 25-30 minutes or until the top becomes slightly browned.

10. The cauliflower buns are best served hot right out of the oven. They do not refrigerate or re-heat well (they will get mushy), but they are so delicious that you'll no doubt eat them right away!

Cranberry Jalapeño "Cornbread" Muffins

Ingredients

1 cup coconut flour

1/3 cup Swerve Sweetener or another erythritol

1 tbsp baking powder

1/2 tsp salt

7 large eggs, lightly beaten

1 cup unsweetened almond milk

1/2 cup butter, melted OR avocado oil

1/2 tsp vanilla

1 cup fresh cranberries, cut in half

3 tbsp minced jalapeño peppers

1 jalapeño, seeds removed, sliced into 12 slices, for garnish

Instructions

1. Preheat oven to 325F and grease a muffin tin well or line with paper liners.

2. In a medium bowl, whisk together coconut flour, sweetener, baking powder, and salt. Break up any clumps with the back of a fork.

3. Stir in eggs, melted butter, and almond milk and stir vigorously. Stir in vanilla extract and continue to stir until mixture is smooth and well combined. Stir in chopped cranberries and jalapeños.

4. Divide batter evenly among prepared muffin cups and place one slice of jalapeño on top of each.

5. Bake 25 to 30 minutes or until tops are set and a tester inserted in the center comes out clean. Let cool 10 minutes in the pan, then transfer to a wire rack to cool completely.

Recipe Notes

Food energy: 157kcal | Saturated fatty acids: 7.11g | Total fat: 11.22g | Calories from fat: 101 | Cholesterol: 128mg | Carbohydrate: 7.08g | Total dietary fiber: 3.84g | Protein: 5.21g | Sodium: 362mg

Keto Bagel

Ingredients

1 cup (120 g) of almond flour

1/4 cup (28 g) of coconut flour

1 Tablespoon (7 g) of psyllium husk powder

1 teaspoon (2 g) of baking powder

1 teaspoon (3 g) of garlic powder

pinch salt

2 medium eggs (88 g)

2 teaspoons (10 ml) of white wine vinegar

2 1/2 Tablespoons (38 ml) of ghee, melted

1 Tablespoon (15 ml) of olive oil

1 teaspoon (5 g) of sesame seeds

Instructions

1. Preheat the oven to 320°F (160°C).

2. Combine the almond flour, coconut flour, psyllium husk powder, baking powder, garlic powder and salt in a bowl.

3. In a separate bowl, whisk the eggs and vinegar together. Slowly drizzle in the melted ghee (which should not be piping hot) and whisk in well.

4. Add the wet mixture to the dry mixture and use a wooden spoon to combine well. Leave to sit for 2-3 minutes.

5. Divide the mixture into 4 equal-sized portions. Using your hands, shape the mixture into a round shape and place onto a tray lined with parchment paper. Use a small spoon or apple corer to make the center hole.

6. Brush the tops with olive oil and scatter over the sesame seeds. Bake in the oven for 20-25 minutes until cooked through. Allow cooling slightly before enjoying!

Keto Breakfast Pizza

Ingredients:

2 cups grated cauliflower

2 tablespoons coconut flour

1/2 teaspoon salt

4 eggs

1 tablespoon psyllium husk powder (Use a mold-free brand like this one)

Toppings: smoked Salmon, avocado, herbs, spinach, olive oil (see post for more suggestions)

Instructions:

Preheat the oven to 350 degrees. Line a pizza tray or sheet pan with parchment.

In a mixing bowl, add all ingredients except toppings and mix until combined. Set aside for 5 minutes to allow coconut flour and psyllium husk to absorb liquid and thicken up.

Carefully pour the breakfast pizza base onto the pan. Use your hands to mold it into a round, even pizza crust.

Bake for 15 minutes, or until golden brown and fully cooked.

Remove from the oven and top breakfast pizza with your chosen toppings. Serve warm.

Nutritional Information

Calories: 454 | Total Fat: 31g | Saturated Fat: 75g | Cholesterol: 348mg | Total Carbs: 26g | Fiber: 17.2g | Sugars: 4.4g | Net Carbs: 8.8g | Protein: 22g | Sodium: 1,325mg | Potassium: 991mg | Calcium: 235mg | Vitamin D: 35mcg | Iron: 3mg

3 Ingredient Mini Paleo Pizza Bases Crusts

Ingredients

For the coconut flour option

8 large egg whites for thicker bases, use 5 whole eggs and 3 egg whites

1/4 cup coconut flour sifted

1/2 tsp baking powder

Spices of choice salt, pepper, Italian spices

Extra coconut flour to dust very lightly

For the almond flour option

8 large egg whites

1/2 cup almond flour

1/2 tsp baking powder

Spices of choice salt, pepper, Italian spices

For the pizza sauce

1/2 cup Mutti tomato sauce

2 cloves garlic crushed

1/4 tsp sea salt

1 tsp dried basil

Instructions

To make the pizza bases/crusts

1. In a large mixing bowl, whisk the eggs/egg whites until opaque. Sift in the coconut flour or almond flour and whisk very well until clumps are removed. Add the baking powder, mixed spices and continue to whisk until completely combined.

2. On low heat, heat a small pan and grease lightly.

3. Once the frying pan is hot, pour the batter in the pan and ensure it is fully coated. Cover the pan with a lid/tray for 3-4 minutes or until bubbles start to appear on top. Flip, cook for an extra 2 minutes and remove from pan- Keep an eye on this, as it can burn out pretty quickly.

4. Continue until all the batter is used up.

5. Allow pizza bases to cool. Once cool, use a skewer and poke holes roughly over the top, for even cooking. Dust very lightly with a dash of coconut flour.

To make the sauce

Combine all the ingredients and let sit at room temperature for at least 30 minutes- This thickens up.

Notes

For a crispy pizza base, bake in the oven for 3-4 minutes before adding your toppings. If you want to freeze them, allow pizza bases to cool completely before topping with a dash of coconut flour and a thin layer of pizza sauce. Ensure each pizza base is divided with parchment paper before placing in the freezer.

Nutrition

Serving: 1Base | Calories: 125kcal | Carbohydrates: 6g | Protein: 8g | Fat: 1g | Fiber: 3g | Vitamin A: 1% | Vitamin C: 2% | Calcium: 1% | Iron: 2%

Keto Pumpkin Bread

Ingredients

1/2 cup butter, softened

2/3 cup erythritol sweetener, like Swerve

4 eggs large

3/4 cup pumpkin puree, canned (see notes for fresh)

1 tsp vanilla extract

1 1/2 cup almond flour

1/2 cup coconut flour

4 tsp baking powder

1 tsp cinnamon

1/2 tsp nutmeg

1/4 tsp ginger

1/8 tsp cloves

1/2 tsp salt

Instructions

1. Preheat the oven to 350°F. Grease a 9"x5" loaf pan, and line with parchment paper.
2. In a large mixing bowl, cream the butter and sweetener together until light and fluffy.
3. Add the eggs, one at a time, and mix well to combine.
4. Add the pumpkin puree and vanilla, and mix well to combine.
5. In a separate bowl, stir together the almond flour, coconut flour, baking powder, cinnamon, nutmeg, ginger, cloves, salt. Break up any lumps of almond flour or coconut flour.

6. Add the dry ingredients to the wet ingredients, and stir to combine. (Optionally, add up to 1/2 cup of mix-ins, like chopped nuts or chocolate chips.)

7. Pour the batter into the prepared loaf pan. Bake for 45 - 55 minutes, or until a toothpick inserted into the center of the loaf comes out clean.

8. If the bread is browning too quickly, you can cover the pan with a piece of aluminum foil.

Notes

Want to use your own homemade puréed pumpkin? If it's thinner than canned pumpkin, try to remove some of the water to prevent soggy pumpkin bread.

Want cream cheese frosting? Check the post above for an easy cream cheese frosting recipe.

Want some nuts or chocolate chips? Feel free to add 1/2 cup of mix-ins to the batter before baking

Want pumpkin muffins instead? Divide the batter into greased muffin tins. Be sure to reduce the baking time.

Nutrition Information:

Amount Per Serving: Calories: 165 Total Fat: 14g Saturated Fat: 7g Unsaturated Fat: 4g Cholesterol: 99mg Sodium: 76mg Carbohydrates: 6g Fiber: 3g Sugar: 1g Protein: 5g

Low Carb Gluten Free Cranberry Bread

Ingredients

2 cups almond flour

1/2 cup powdered erythritol or Swerve, see Note

1/2 teaspoon Steviva stevia powder see Note

1 1/2 teaspoons baking powder

1/2 teaspoon baking soda

1 teaspoon salt

4 tablespoons unsalted butter melted (or coconut oil)

1 teaspoon blackstrap molasses optional (for brown sugar flavor)

4 large eggs at room temperature

1/2 cup coconut milk

1 bag cranberries 12 ounces

Instructions

1. Preheat oven to 350 degrees; grease a 9-by-5 inch loaf pan and set aside.
2. In a large bowl, whisk together flour, erythritol, stevia, baking powder, baking soda, and salt; set aside.
3. In a medium bowl, combine butter, molasses, eggs, and coconut milk.
4. Mix dry mixture into the wet mixture until well combined.
5. Fold in cranberries. Pour batter into prepared pan.
6. Bake until a toothpick inserted in the center of the loaf comes clean, about 1 hour and 15 minutes.

7. Transfer pan to a wire rack; let the bread cool 15 minutes before removing from pan.

8. Notes

9. Sweeteners can be replaced with about 3/4 to 1 cup of any low carb sugar replacement depending on sweetness desired.

Cinnamon Almond Flour Bread

Ingredients

2 cups fine blanched almond flour (I use Bob's, Red Mill)

2 tbsp coconut flour

1/2 tsp sea salt

1 tsp baking soda

1/4 cup Flaxseed meal or chia meal (ground chia or flaxseed, see notes for how to make your own)

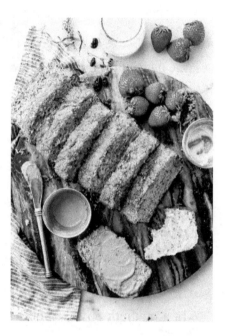

5 Eggs and 1 egg white whisked together

1.5 tsp Apple cider vinegar or lemon juice

2 tbsp maple syrup or honey

2–3 tbsp of clarified butter (melted) or Coconut oil; divided. Vegan butter also works

1 tbsp cinnamon plus extra for topping

Optional chia seed to sprinkle on top before baking

Instructions

1. Preheat oven to 350F. Line an 8×4 bread pan with parchment paper at the bottom and grease the sides.

2. In a large bowl, mix your almond flour, coconut flour, salt, baking soda, flaxseed meal or chia meal, and 1/2 tablespoon of cinnamon.

3. In another small bowl, whisk together your eggs and egg white. Then add in your maple syrup (or honey), apple cider vinegar, and melted butter (1.5 to 2 tbsp).

4. Mix wet ingredients into dry. Be sure to remove any clumps that might have occurred from the almond flour or coconut flour.

5. Pour batter into your greased loaf pan.

6. Bake at 350° for 30-35 minutes, until a toothpick inserted into the center of the loaf comes out clean. Mine too around 35 minutes but I am at altitude.

7. Remove from and oven.

8. Next, whisk together the other 1 to 2 tbsp of melted butter (or oil) and mix it with 1/2 tbsp of cinnamon. Brush this on top of your cinnamon almond flour bread.

9. Cool and serve or store for later.